AF477178

A Textbook of Pharmacy Practice

A TEXTBOOK OF PHARMACY PRACTICE

Prof. S. Balasubramanian
M.Pharm.
C. L. Baid Metha College of Pharmacy, Chennai.
Former Principal, College of Allied Medical Sciences, Madurai and
Professor, St.Jhon College of Pharmacy, Warangal, Telangana.

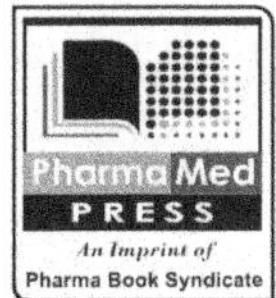

PharmaMed Press

An imprint of Pharma Book Syndicate
A unit of BSP Books Pvt. Ltd.
4-4-309/316, Giriraj Lane,
Sultan Bazar, Hyderabad - 500 095.

Published by

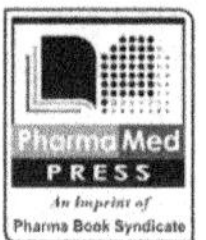

PharmaMed Press

An imprint of Pharma Book Syndicate
A unit of BSP Books Pvt. Ltd.
4-4-309/316, Giriraj Lane, Sultan Bazar, Hyderabad - 500 095.
Phone: 040-23445600, 23445688; Fax: 91+40-23445611
E-mail: info@pharmamedpress.com
www.pharmamedpress.com/pharmamedpress.net

ISBN: 978-93-89974-38-6

Dedicated to the Memory of my Better Half

Mrs. M. Chellam Balasubramanian

PREFACE

The book 'Pharmacy Practice' in your hand is the culmination of the long experience of the author as a practicing pharmacist as well as the pharmacy teacher. It is written in accordance with the new syllabus framed by the Pharmacy Council of India for the semester pattern of the undergraduate course in pharmacy.

A student who wishes to practice as a hospital or community pharmacist should acquire working knowledge by mastering the subject matters of the book. All the fundamental requirements for the same are described in relevant chapters. Illustrations and examples are given wherever necessary.

The pharmacy practice of the modern world has changed from product-oriented to patient-oriented long back in developed countries. India is yet to pick-up the concept. Nevertheless, it is on the horizon after the introduction of the 6-year Pharm.D course in India for whom also this book will be useful to a certain extent.

Finally, I wish to record my gratitude to the management of my present and former institutions for their support and wonderful collection of resources in their libraries for reference. I also appreciate the publishers M/s BSP Books Private limited, Hyderabad for bringing out this book in such a nice manner.

-Prof. S. Balasubramanian

Chennai.

CONTENTS

CHAPTER 6

Hospital Formulary

CHAPTER 7

Therapeutic Drug Monitoring

CHAPTER 8

Medication Adherence

CHAPTER 9

Patient Medication History Interview

CHAPTER 10

Community Pharmacy Management

CHAPTER 11

Pharmacy and Therapuetics Committee

CHAPTER 12

Drug Information Services and Poison Information Centre

CHAPTER 13

Patient Counseling

CHAPTER 14

Education and Training Program in the Hospital

CHAPTER 15

Prescribed Medication Order and Communication Skills

CHAPTER 16

Budget Preparation and Implementation

CHAPTER 17

Clinical Pharmacy

CHAPTER 18

Over the Counter (OTC) Sales

CHAPTER 19

Drug Store Management and Inventory Control

CHAPTER 20

Investigational use of Drugs

CHAPTER 21

Interpretation of Clinical Laboratory Tests

CHAPTER 1

HOSPITAL AND ITS ORGANIZATION

LEARNING OBJECTIVE

On completion of this chapter, the student should be able to explain the organizational structure and functions of a hospital, its types and human resources. The understanding of the function and structure of a hospital will be useful for him to start his carrier as a hospital pharmacist.

DEFINITION

Hospital is an organization and institution of public health and welfare. It provides healthcare facilities to ensure the well-being of people through specialized equipment handled by a group of specially trained individuals. Contrary to the common perception, a hospital not only takes care of sick people, it is also responsible for keeping a check on the well-being and maintaining health standards of the people in general. In order to keep them disease-free and in good health, a hospital undertakes immunization, runs educational programs to spread information regarding personal and social hygienic practices.

Classification

Hospitals can be classified both on the clinical basis and non-clinical basis. The former classification may be either on the criteria of the system of treatment followed in a particular hospital or on the basis of specialization of a particular disease or part of the human body. On the other hand, the non-clinical method of classification is based on other general parameters. For instance, the classification can be done based on size, facilities offered, or ownership of the hospital.

To wrap up, hospitals can be classified based on the following criteria:

I. Size and Facilities

II. Ownership

III. System of treatment and

IV. Specialization.

I. Size

More conveniently, hospitals are classified on the basis of the size, that is the number of beds available for patients that it can intake and treat. There can be hospitals with following bed capacity and hence, they lie under categories.

A. Less than 20 beds

B. Between 20 to 100 beds and

C. Above 100 beds (up to 1000 and more)

As mentioned above, the hospitals are also classified according to the facilities they offer and based on that, there are three major categories: Primary, Secondary and Tertiary hospitals. They can also be referred to as small, medium and large hospitals. Many hospitals run by private practitioners fall under the first category of small hospitals. These usually have one or two general wards available for the patients.

Furthermore, there might be only a couple of doctors working here and these hospitals may not have several diagnostic facilities like clinical lab, x-ray, scan, etc. They refer their patients to third-party agencies for these services. Primary health centers (PHC) run by government can be classified under this category and they are all aptly called as primary care hospitals, where the majority of patients go to get treatment for their illness. Many of these hospitals are not open during the night time.

Medium sized hospitals are those operating in small towns like Taluk headquarters. Here, an approximate of 5 to 10 doctors may be working that also includes a couple of specialists. These hospitals also offer some of the diagnostic facilities. The cases that are beyond the working module of primary level hospitals are sent to these secondary care hospitals for treatment. In a few essential wards like a medical ward, surgical ward, pediatric ward, and maternity ward, up to 100 beds are available in these hospitals. These hospitals are operational during day and night alike.

Large hospitals are highly specialized healthcare institutions with almost all medical facilities available to the patients. Their bed strength ranges from 100 to 1000. The district headquarters hospitals, Teaching (Medical College) hospitals and most of the giant private, corporate hospitals fall under this category. They are also called as tertiary hospitals or referral hospitals because more complicated cases from the first two types of hospitals are referred here for further treatment. Usually, an estimate of more than 50 doctors and over 300 Paramedical professionals work in these hospitals in 3 shifts throughout the day.

II. Ownership

Hospitals can also be classified according to ownership. There are two broader categories for this type:

1. Government-owned hospitals and 2. Private hospitals

1. Government Hospitals

From Primary Health Centers in small villages to Taluk, District, and Medical college hospitals in cities, a large number of hospitals are owned by the state governments. Additionally, there are several quasi/semi-government hospitals that are going by different names like local body hospitals like municipal hospitals, (municipal) corporation hospitals and panchayat union hospitals. These are run by local bodies which get financial aid from the government to serve the purpose.

On a much larger scale, Central Government also owns some hospitals like the Central Government Health Scheme (CGHS) hospitals, All India Institute of Medical Sciences (AIIMS), etc. Some of these hospitals are run by the central government undertakings or corporations to serve a particular group of people like railway hospitals, port trust hospitals, military hospitals, ESI hospital, etc.

2. Private Hospitals

There are many private hospitals of the same size, if not bigger than the Government hospitals. They are established by trusts, societies, families, and even resourceful individuals. They are well-equipped with specialized medical equipment, facilities and doctors with different specializations. They are also called corporate hospitals. For instance, Apollo Group of Hospitals is one such hospital chain. Medium and small private hospitals are available in all the cities and towns of our country. These private hospitals offer facilities and standards that are on par with that of the Western countries, thereby attracting a lot of patients from abroad to come to India for medical treatment at very nominal expenses (medical tourism).

III.   System of Treatment

These groups of hospitals are those in which different systems are followed for treatment. They are Ayurveda Hospitals, Siddha Hospitals, Unani Hospitals or Homeopathy Hospitals. The physicians in these hospitals are well-educated and/ or have experience in these specific methods of treatment. They use the medicines specific to these systems or methods for treatment. These hospitals or physicians are popular in rural areas because they have marked their existence even before the allopathic system of treatment was introduced by British Rulers in our country.

IV.   Specialization Basis

Hospitals can also be classified according to the specialized services offered in a particular hospital. For example, there are a few hospitals which only treat a particular part of the body or a particular disease. Thus, we have two groups:

Group I

A. Eye hospital

B. Dental hospital

C. ENT hospital

D. Chest hospital and

E. Skin hospital

Group II

(i)   Psychiatric hospital

(ii) Orthopedics hospital and

(iii) Communicable and infectious diseases hospital.

All this apart, there are some other hospitals that offer treatment to a special group of patients like Children's Hospital, Maternity hospital, etc. In all these hospitals, doctors who are qualified in particular specialization are employed.

Thus, in a big country like India, there is a multiple variety of hospitals and practices followed for medical treatment. The Government of India has recently brought legislation, by name, Clinical Establishments Registration act, which envisage registration of all types of hospitals and clinics in the country. Hence, they can also be classified according to the facilities available in them into Grade I, II, III, etc.

ORGANIZATION

The nature and size of the organization of a hospital differ according to the requirement. The organization of a big hospital has two separate wings, one for the clinical administration and the other for office administration. The structure of these wings is given below:

The clinical administration and office administration both have multiple divisions or departments and every section is headed by a qualified person with specialization and experience in the particular subject. Needless to point out, large administrative bodies require individuals with special training and education in hospital administration.

Medium size hospitals like the Taluk hospitals and the ones in small towns differ when it comes to organizational setup. As already mentioned some of the sections/wings may not be available in these hospitals. They are added whenever necessary. Because these hospitals are too big to be managed by an individual, the Government or trust forms various committees to assist the Deans in their administration.

These committees are called Governing councils or Board of Directors. They have members from the trust and various departments of the hospital and even people from outside. People's representatives like MLA, MLC, MP or MC are often given membership in Government Hospital Councils to function effectively and to meet the medical requirements of the people.

Apart from this, various subcommittees are also formed at various levels of the hospital for the same reason e.g.: Finance committee, purchase committee, development committee, ethical committee, etc. Thus, big hospitals are well- organized and function smoothly.

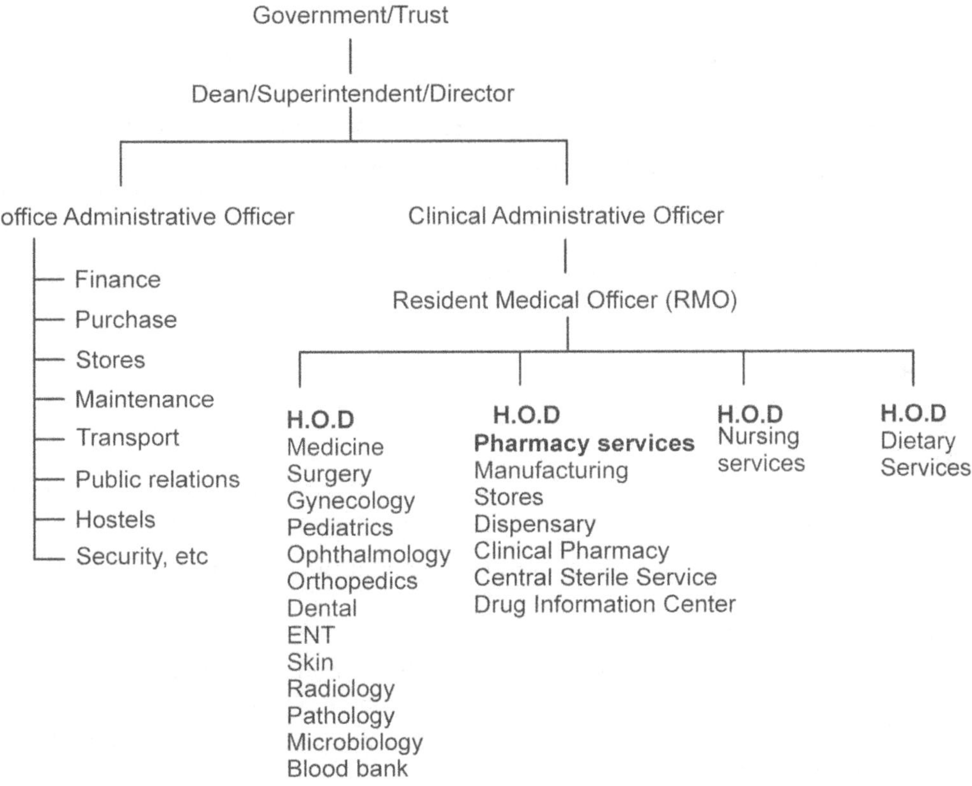

Flow chart of a Hospital Organization

Administration

The above committees regularly conduct meetings and forward their recommendations to the Governing Council or Board of Directors, where these recommendations are considered, approved, modified or rejected. The approved decisions are then implemented by the Deans, either through their office administrative or clinical administrative wing.

Only policy matters and/or the decisions involving a huge sum of money are thus routed through the governing council. While the other small issues and day to day affairs are decided by the Deans themselves and implemented accordingly. However, Deans report all the important matters to the Council or Trust or Government through on a periodic basis.

Functions

The major functions of a hospital are,

1. Treatment of patients

2. Prevention of diseases and

3. Education of public

As pointed out above, hospitals are not only treating the patients but also preventing the disease from occurring and spreading. They undertake large scale immunization programs by vaccination drives and other programs like oral polio drop campaign, health camps to identify and prevent diseases in a particular area or demographic. As we know, prevention is better than cure, the Government of India gives more importance to these health related drives and programs. Many public health programs like mosquito eradication, chlorination of drinking water, etc, are promoted through various Government bodies.

To carry out all the above functions, various categories of personnel are employed in hospitals which are described below:

Medical Staff and their Duties

As already given in the organizational structure of the hospital, there are scores of medical and paramedical departments in a hospital. For all practical purposes, both these departments can be referred to as medical departments, as there are a significant number of non-medical staff working in any hospital who are not directly involved in the treatment of patients.

Medical staff list of the hospital starts from the top administer -- the dean or superintendent or director of the hospital and goes on to include HODs, Surgeons, Assistant surgeons, and House surgeon, who are listed at the bottom of the hierarchy. Similarly, there are a number of individuals heading the departments of non-medical and Paramedics, with junior pharmacists, nursing orderly or Lab technicians working according to the authorities they have in these departments. They all work in coordination with the sole aim of giving the best treatment to the patients coming to the hospital.

If it is a teaching or a medical college hospital, senior doctors teach the medical students during and after the hospital hours. They teach by demonstrating the conditions of patients that come to the hospitals and also via lectures in medical colleges in the afternoons.

Among all the departments, medical and surgical departments hold the major share of functions and responsibilities of the hospital. The concerning medical professionals first attend to the patients in the out-patient department and either start the treatment right away or refer the patient to other specialization departments like skin, Gynecology, etc. If required, they admit the patient in the wards. After conducting the required diagnostic tests, the prescription is given if it is an outpatient or documented in the case sheets of in-patients in the ward. This is done after the OP hours during the ward rounds. After performing similar tasks in the surgery department, surgeons perform surgeries programmed for the day. These patients are then transferred to the post-operative wards. There, they are taken care of until complete recovery or whenever they are fit enough for discharge. Thus, treating outpatients in OPD, inpatients in the wards, performing surgeries, and other clinical procedures are the routine functions of the medical staff. That apart, they attend to the administrative functions of the hospital and all the important meetings of staff or management.

Most of the time, junior staff of both medical and non-medical departments work during the night shifts and seek the help of the senior staff if required during the functional hours. Occasionally, staff also perform special tasks assigned to them like organizing and conducting medical camps in villages. They also organize and attend seminars and conferences in their fields of specialization.

While performing all these functions, Paramedical staff are contributing their expertise routinely. Nurses take care of inpatients in the wards; administer drugs to patients both in OPD and wards. Pharmacists procure and keep the required drugs ready, dispense them to patients and perform the clinical pharmacy services [as described in a separate chapter later in the book]. Physiotherapists offer required therapy to the patients which are referred to them and the lab technologists help the doctor by performing diagnostic tests prescribed for a patient and their work is complemented by Radiology technicians in x-ray, scan, etc. Dieticians order and supervise the preparation and distribution of nutritious food required for all inpatients and also advises the food regimen to be followed by selected outpatients. All the staff members of the hospital work as a team and ensure that the patient is cured as early as possible and thus, the disease is contained and not allowed to spread or damage the society. That's why the medical profession is called a noble profession by the people.

In order to achieve the aim of 'Health for all', prevention and treatment alone are not sufficient unless the general public is aware and cooperative with the medical schemes. Hence, large scale education campaign is carried out to create awareness among people about diseases, preventive methods, nutrition, and personal and social hygienic practices via multiple communication methods like posters, cinema, TV and other media by the hospital and public health authorities.

QUESTIONS

1. Define hospitals.

2. Draw a flow chart of Hospital Administration.

3. What are secondary care hospitals?

4. What is the significance of the term referral in referral hospitals?

5. Classify hospitals and explain each one of them in detail.

6. What are the functions of a hospital? Explain.

7. How are big hospitals administered? Enumerate the role of various committees formed in hospitals.

8. Explain the functions of Medical staff of a hospital.

Chapter **2**

HOSPITAL PHARMACY AND ITS ORGANIZATION

LEARNING OBJECTIVE

This chapter will enlighten the students about hospital pharmacy organization, its location and layout, various sections, technocrats employed, functions and role and responsibilities of a hospital pharmacist. Though the concept of hospital pharmacy is very old, it is yet to take root in India, hence a theoretical knowledge, in the absence of practical acquaintance will be useful to the students and that is the learning objective of elaborate coverage of the chapter.

DEFINITION

"Hospital pharmacy is an organ of a hospital, where drugs are manufactured and/or purchased, stored, dispensed and its uses monitored and also, drug information, education and training are provided to inpatients, outpatients as well as to fellow health professionals by a team of highly qualified pharmacists".

Origin and Development

Long ago, a pharmacy inside the hospital was called 'Hospital Pharmacy', just like a pharmacy among the community is called 'Community Pharmacy'. These pharmacies have merely managed the job of 'dispensing drugs' to the patients coming with a prescription.

However, a modern 'Hospital Pharmacy' is very different from these. Its services are broader and serve the entire range of purposes with respect to the drugs. From dispensing to Therapeutic Drug Monitoring (TDM), a modern pharmacist is expected to perform all the services involving drugs at the patient level. Earlier, the responsibilities of a pharmacist were limited to only dispensing the drugs but now these are followed by other important services like the clinical pharmacy services, A pharmacist also has to obtain medication history of the patient, advice the doctors in selecting suitable drugs for the patient, monitor the therapy, intervene if necessary to correct the course of treatment and offer counselling to the patient either during treatment or at the time of discharge.

Thus, objectives and functions of hospital pharmacy and its organization have widened enormously owing to its transformation from product-oriented service to patient-oriented service.

But at the outset, one must be clear that in India the above-mentioned modern hospital pharmacy services are not currently available in all the hospitals. However, there are a few exemptions like Christian Medical College Hospital, Vellore in Tamil Nadu and Trivandrum Medical College Hospital, Thiruvananthapuram. Nevertheless, these services have to be introduced sooner or later in India, as and when people realize their rights and requirements.

Hence, a pharmacy student should study about this ideal hospital pharmacy set up and be familiarized with its requirements and services expected from them. They must strive to achieve this in their own interest as well as that of the society they live in.

The following pages describe the ideal hospital pharmacy set up to be established in India. These are well along on the lines of the ones that already exist in the developed countries.

Organizational Structure

The organizational set-up of a hospital pharmacy starts with a fully qualified and experienced Head of the Department. They must have the necessary education, specialization, training, and experience in the majority of the functions of a Hospital Pharmacy. Thus, an M.Pharm graduate with Ph.D. and specialization either in Pharmacology, Pharmacy Practice or Clinical Pharmacy is a suitable candidate for the job. Alternatively, a 'Pharm D' graduate with a relevant experience in the field is also apt for the job as these graduates have adequate exposure in the hospital. It is important to note that they are given preference over the others in western and developed countries.

The head of the department is accompanied by various section heads with experience in the relevant fields of specialization. For example, pharmacy postgraduates and graduates with experience and endorsement by the Drugs Control Administration are appointed in the drugs manufacturing sections of the Hospital Pharmacy.

Similarly, pharmacy graduates with experience in the analysis and quality control of drugs and formulations are given charge of the quality control section.

Furthermore, the medical stores of the hospital are run by pharmacy graduates with experience in dispensing drugs. In both these sections, D. Pharm holders are also appointed in adequate numbers to help with the tasks.

The Central Sterile Service Department of the hospital, which supplies the required material in sterile conditions to various departments, is also headed by pharmacy graduates assisted by D. Pharm holders.

Once dispensing is over, clinical pharmacy services commence. These are highly skilled and professional services which are also referred to as 'Pharmaceutical Care'. Going by the exact definition, it is the responsible provision of drug therapy for the purpose of achieving definite outcomes that improves the quality of life of the patient. The success of pharmaceutical care lies in determining or anticipating drug-related problems and taking measures to improve outcomes. Thereby, it results in a better quality of life for the patients. Hence, this section of hospital pharmacy requires highly qualified pharmacist with relevant experience. For this section, M. Pharm graduates in pharmacology, clinical pharmacy or pharmacy practice specialization or Pharm. D graduates are appointed. Additionally, adequate numbers of assistants are provided to carry out the enormous tasks involved.

The remaining services of a hospital pharmacy like Drug Information Services, Education and Training, etc. are also suitably manned by appointing pharmacy professionals with relevant qualification and experience in the field. Thus, an organization of a modern 'Hospital Pharmacy' consists of at least 9 sections as described below in the form of a flow chart.

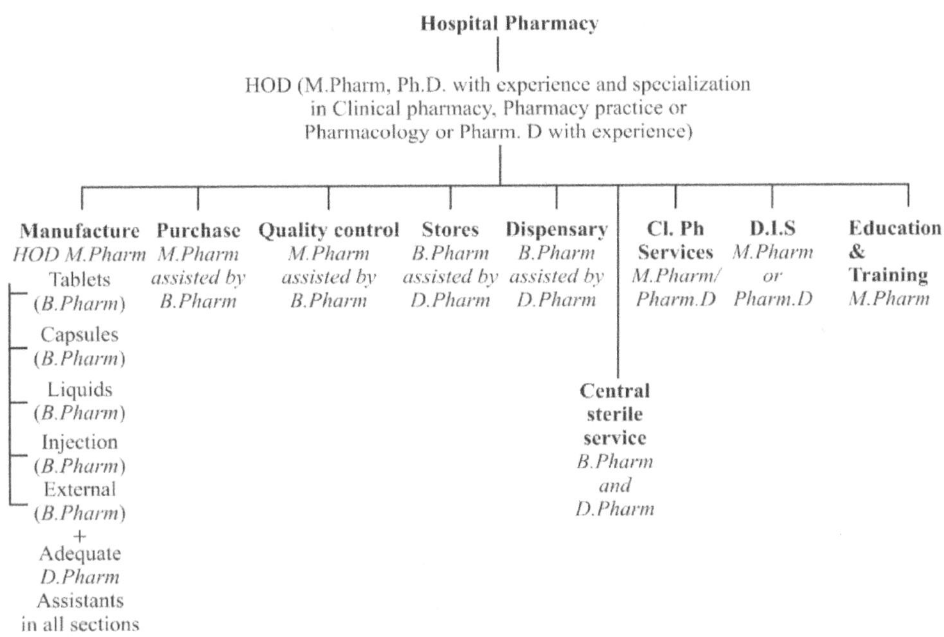

Flow Chart of a Modern Hospital Pharmacy Organization

Location and Layout

As per the above organizational structure, an ideal hospital pharmacy department should have nine sections. Needless to mention, that all these sections may not necessarily exist at a single location. Depending upon the services provided, they should be at apt places, making it convenient and trouble free for the patients, visitors, and staff working in the particular section.

A dispensary must be near the exit point of the hospital so that the out-patients can collect their medicines and move out of the hospital without disturbing the in-patients. On the other hand, the Drug Information Center [DIC] require a calm and quiet place where visitors, students, and scholars can read and get any information they need without having to be disturbed by the hospital chaos. Moreover, the Education and training services should be near

DIC as they require books, journals, and other educational tools to serve the purpose. A couple of classrooms or seminar halls can co-exist in this area for similar reasons. Drug stores and purchase sections can be located in the same building so that their quick and hassle-free coordination can be ensured. Central sterile service department needs to be near the main operation theaters but need not be on the same floor of the building. Also, clinical pharmacists should be given cabins near the wards they are posted.

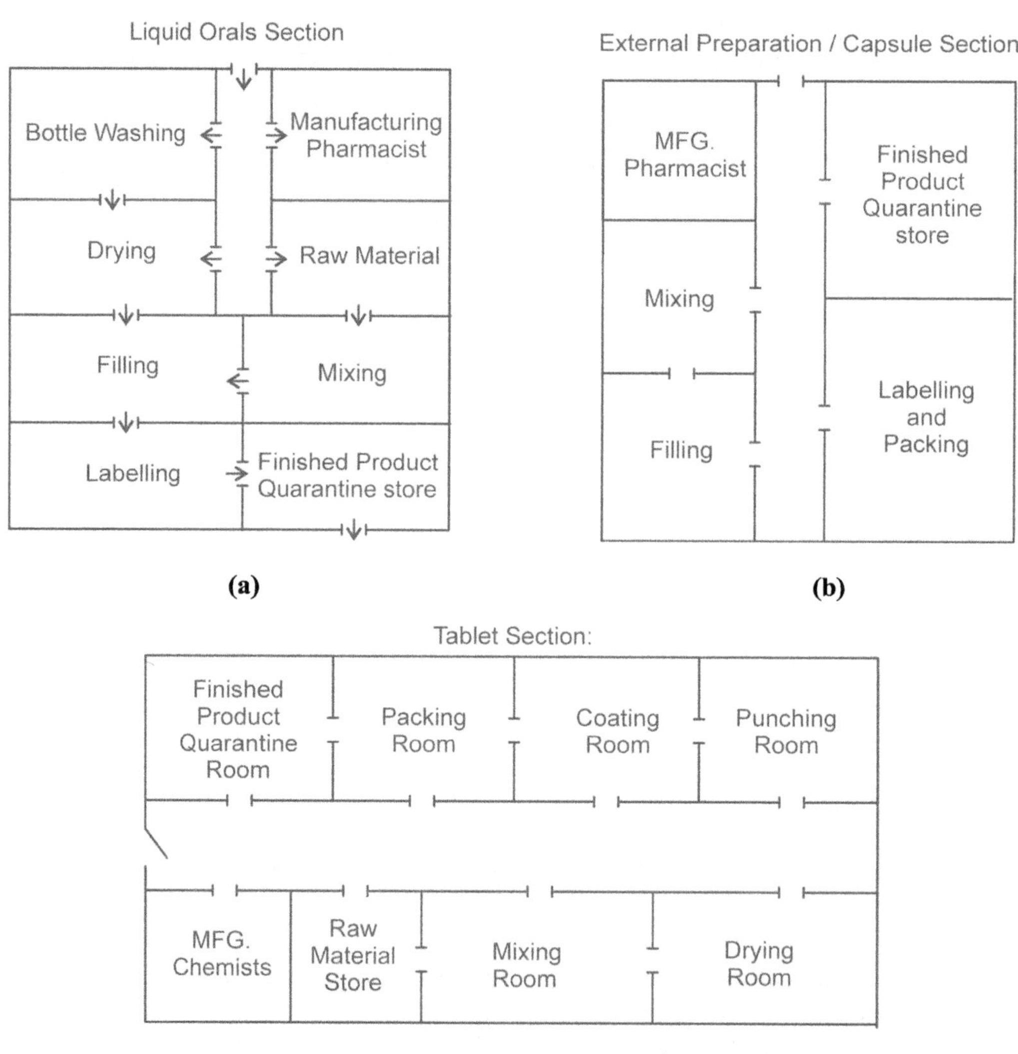

Injection Section:

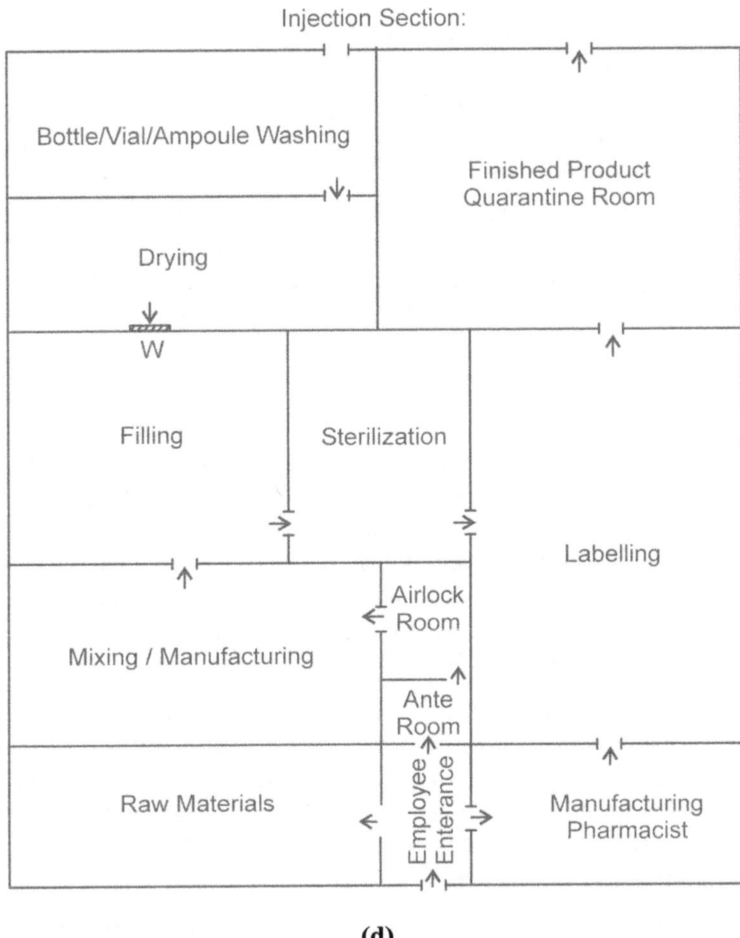

(d)

Finally, if the manufacturing of drugs is undertaken inside a particular hospital, it only makes sense to keep it away from the wards as it is set to function like a factory. As any manufacturing facility requires movement of men, machine and materials on a daily basis, a careful layout planning is of utmost priority. Needless to mention, the manufacturing facility should be accompanied by a quality control section as per the law. In order to coordinate all these sections, the office of the head of the department of pharmacy should be located in the administrative block of the hospital with appropriate internal and external communication facilities. Here, the layout plan for manufacturing section is given for reference. But all the other sections can be established by the hospital management, keeping in mind the requirements pointed out above.

Staff and Infrastructure

Staff: From the above organizational flow chart, we can easily list the number of staff required for a modern hospital pharmacy. It is not hard to comprehend that this number depends on the workload or the amount of activities carried out in each section of the Hospital Pharmacy.

Hence, the first and the foremost thing before settling on the number of people required is to fix the services which the hospital pharmacy intends to provide.

In a full-fledged hospital pharmacy like the one charted above, there are nine mandatory sections that should capacitate people with a specialization or experience in the relevant area. Thus, starting with director or HOD of the Hospital Pharmacy, it is important that these sections are headed by experienced people. The director or HOD of the hospital pharmacy must have the overall knowledge of each section of their department. Hence, an M.Pharm, Ph.D. or Pharm.D with minimum 10 years experience in various pharmacy-related tasks would be an ideal person for the job. They are supported by a few associates, deputy directors with the same qualifications but less experience (5-6 years).

The manufacturing section of the hospital pharmacy not only requires experience but also an approval or eligibility to get approval from the Drugs Control Department for the manufacture of the formulation concerned. Similarly, the quality control section where the hospital manufactured or procured drugs are tested for quality should have experienced and approved analytical pharmacists. They should be able to independently handle and operate intricate modern analytical instruments and equipment. Furthermore, pharmacists with experience in the manufacture and analysis of injectable, especially in Large Volume Parenterals [LVP] play an important role in the hospital pharmacy manufacturing units as these LVPs are the single largest drug used daily in almost all the wards of the hospitals.

Moving on to the next important section of a hospital pharmacy which is clinical pharmacy services section. Here pharmacists can provide advisory and consultancy services to the treating physicians, Hence, Pharm.D graduates with experience must be appointed in this section. The clinical pharmacists also have to perform the patients' medication history interview, therapeutic drug monitoring and counseling in this section. Hence, Pharm.D or M.Pharm Pharmacy Practice graduates should be trained for the said job in this area.

The other sections like medical and surgical stores, purchase, dispensary, central sterile service, and drug information center should be provided with regular staff with relevant experience. Education and a training section, on the other hand, requires a well-experienced staff.

In conclusion, all sections of a hospital pharmacy should be manned with suitable pharmacists, this process is easier said than done. Hence, the manpower requirement of the hospital pharmacy should be thoroughly studied and planned accordingly. Getting experienced people for each section can be a tough task. So, it becomes important that a suitable training program should be developed where recent/fresh pharmacy graduates are recruited as 'Resident pharmacists' similar to Resident Doctors or 'House Surgeons' of the medical field. These resident pharmacists should be appointed in all the sections of hospital pharmacy in rotation where seniors in the field are available to train, supervise and evaluate their work. Thus, suitable manpower can be created in the due course of time.

Infrastructure

In order to provide proper and effective service to the patients, a good infrastructure is a must for the hospital pharmacy. These infrastructure facilities can be as per the following requirements:

(a) All the equipment and instruments for the manufacture and analysis of formulation as per schedule M for Drugs and Cosmetics acts and rules of Govt of India. They are required to follow GMP and GLP as per WHO and USFDA standards.

(b) All the necessary equipment for compounding, repacking and dispensing in the main, satellite and ward pharmacies should be according to the medical and pharmacy manuals and orders of the government.

(c) There must be proper storage facilities including refrigerators, air conditioners, cupboards, storage space, floor space and lightings in the medical and surgical stores of the hospital. These stores as well as dispensaries should have separate cupboards with lock facilities for narcotics and other controlled substances.

(d) Central sterile service section should be equipped with the latest sterilization facilities and storage area must be free from contamination with laminar workbench, airlock, etc.

(e) All these areas must be provided with uninterrupted power supply using generators, invertors, etc in order to ensure smooth and hassle-free processing and storing of drugs.

(f) A library with latest books and online database resources should be available for use by pharmacists and doctors alike. There should be necessary facilities for data retrieval, storage, copying, and recording. The latest editions of "Pharmacopoeias, a textbook on pharmacology, along with textbooks for toxicology, therapeutics biochemistry, microbiology, drugs indexes, professional periodicals (journals) on the above subjects must be available in the library at all times..

(g) In order to maintain the above facilities, adequate clerical and non-clerical STAFF should be provided. Hence, a well-equipped office with stenographic, bookkeeping people must be available. Additionally, the furniture and fixtures necessary for all the above activities must be in place.

Functions

As described in the flow chart above, each section of the modern hospital pharmacy performs specific functions assigned which are described below:

1. Manufacturing Section

(i) Estimate the annual demand for each drug used in the hospital.

(ii) Plan the production schedule.

(iii) Manufacture the required items after procuring the necessary raw materials, packing materials, etc.

(iv) Carry out any special work entrusted to it like preparation of IV admixture, total parenteral nutrition, etc.

(v) Check the standards of formulations as set by QC and QA department.

2. Purchase Section

(i)   Estimate the demand or the quantity of drug required.

(ii)   Set up the specifications for the needed drugs that arrive, in consultation with the departments concerned. This includes quality, quantity, packing, strength, etc.

(iii) Follow the approved purchase procedure like calling for tenders, quotations, and identifying the suppliers to place orders.

(iv)   Receive, verify and dispatch the drugs to a quarantine area and then to the stores after approval by the quality control section.

(v)   Settle the bills and be ready for any emergency purchases.

3. Quality Control Section

(i)   Prepare the methods of analysis, equipment, chemicals and other requirements for almost all drugs either manufactured or purchased by the hospital.

(ii)   Draw samples from the manufacturing section or quarantine area if purchased from outside.

(iii) Analyze and submit reports to the people concerned. Thus, certifying the quality of drugs used in the hospital.

(iv)   Undertake research and development studies with respect to the drugs manufactured in the hospital in order to improve its efficacy as well as to reduce the cost.

(v)   Send samples to third-party laboratories, if required.

4. Stores Section

(i)   Receives drugs from either manufacturing section or purchase department.

(ii)   Store them properly until issued to the dispensary and other places according to specified storage conditions so as to preserve its efficacy and potency.

(iii) Issue drugs to the dispensary and other departments as per their approved indents.

(iv)   Keep an account for all input and output as well as stock on hand (inventory control).

(v)   Monitor the drug use pattern to inform and assist the authorities and manufacturing section in the production plan or purchase plan.

(vi)   Look for the expiry dates of all items stored, periodically and physically. This is followed by bringing to the notice of people concerned about short expiry items so that they can be either used earlier or return to the supplier.

5. Dispensary

(i)   Receive the drugs required for dispensing to outpatients in sufficient quantities from the stores of the hospital.

(ii)   Re-package and Pre-package drugs for dispensing.

(iii) Dispense them to patients while following high standards like auxiliary labels, proper packing, and instructions written on the envelope apart from clear and louder oral instructions.

(iv) Maintain account for the drugs issued on a daily basis.

(v) Provide a clean, neat and comfortable environment for the patients waiting to get their drugs.

6. Central Sterile Supply Department

(i) Procure, install and maintain all the required sterilization equipment.

(ii) Prepare, update, stock and maintain an inventory of items, equipment, and instruments required by various departments of the hospital.

(iii) Sterilize the required items as per the SOP prepared earlier and supply to the departments in need.

(iv) Prepare and circulate educative literature to all the departments concerned on infection control as well as on the maintenance of sterility and sterile area up keeping.

(v) Always keep ready emergency ward supplies.

7. Clinical Pharmacy Services

(i) Engage adequate numbers of clinical pharmacists wherever needed including the outpatient department and all wards.

(ii) Conduct medication history interview for patients admitted in the hospital and forward the relevant details to the treating physician or surgeon.

(iii) Identify the drugs brought to the hospital by the patients and offer guidance on using or discarding them. In any other case, forward the details to the doctor.

(iv) After diagnosis, the clinical pharmacist is required to give his expert opinion on the suitable drug formulation and dose for the particular patient to the treating doctor, if solicited.

(v) Once the treatment commences, they have to monitor the patient for the effects of drugs by conducting necessary pharmacokinetic tests on blood, body fluids and other samples. Based on these tests, they can recommend the doctor to change the medicine, alter the dose or stop the medicine altogether. Adverse drug reactions are particularly monitored on the patients who are on long time treatment.

(vi) They also have to counsel the patients as and when necessary during the course of treatment or at the time of discharge from the hospital. In addition to this, also provide the patients with necessary medicines and instructions to follow to continue the treatment or during home recovery.

(vii) Receive and maintain the feedback sent by patients after discharge.

8. Drug Information Services

(i) Pharmacist in charge of this service is required to collect, arrange and provide the necessary drug information required by the public, health care professionals, and research students.

(ii) Periodically, update the information available.

(iii) Prepare and circulate literature, brochures, bulletins, and circulars on all important matters concerning drug use to all the people involved in the process.

9. Education and Training Services

(i) Provide education and training to student pharmacists, student nurses, student doctors and even to other health care employees of the hospital.

(ii) Undertake educational programs for the public.

(iii) Accept and deliver lectures in professional associations and other clubs like Lions club, Rotary club, etc on the drug-related matters and also on public health issues.

Role and Responsibilities of a Hospital Pharmacist

Earlier, the primary role of a hospital pharmacist was limited to dispensing drugs to the outpatients. This was the major and the only role played by them in a traditional set up until a few decades ago. But after the evolution of the concept of modern hospital pharmacy, their roles have diversified. Now, a modern hospital pharmacist has to take care of the manufacturing and analysis of drug formulations, provide clinical pharmacy services to patients, educate and train student pharmacists, nurses, doctors, provide drug information to medical practitioners, research scholars and the general public. Furthermore, procure, store and distribute drugs, surgical items, and sterile equipment to the operation theaters through central sterile services.

Though all these roles are assigned to hospital pharmacists, in practice, many of these roles are still denied to them in the developing countries. However, today's budding pharmacists may have to shoulder these roles and responsibilities sooner or later once our governments decide to go for full-fledged hospital pharmacy.

Responsibilities of Hospital Pharmacists

(a) Chief pharmacist: They are responsible for the overall functioning of the department. Hence, they must have working knowledge about each and every section of their department and that is why only experienced pharmacists are promoted and appointed as chief pharmacists. A highly academically qualified pharmacist without relevant experience in the said field cannot be directly appointed to the post as they cannot do justice to the post.

The chief pharmacist has the responsibility to plan, organize and control all activities of the hospital pharmacy. They should be able to guide, motivate and supervise the tasks carried out by all the sections of the hospital pharmacy. As they are included as a member of several hospital committees, they are expected to participate and contribute meaningfully to the functions of those committees.

Manufacturing of drug formulations require constant supervision and vigilance on the part of higher authorities. A simple mistake can lead to huge losses and problems to the hospital. So, it is important that these facilities must be thoroughly inspected, often without prior intimation. The chief pharmacist also has similar responsibilities in the proper functioning of central sterile services, clinical pharmacy services, and dispensary. All these services have a great impact on the functioning of various departments of hospitals and in patient safety, and in turn, their satisfaction about pharmacy services.

The chief pharmacist is also responsible for organizing training for pharmacy students and staff. They should organize and participate in public health camps periodically whenever required. Additionally, they should publish newsletters, bulletins, etc. and also maintain a cordial relationship with the other HODs to ensure the smooth functioning of the hospital.

(b)   **Other pharmacists:** The responsibilities of other pharmacists are given above under the heading functions of different sections of hospital pharmacy. One important responsibility common to all these pharmacists is to learn the works of other sections as well. This helps to ensure uninterrupted functioning of the department in case of transfer or emergency. It is also mandatory for the senior pharmacists in charge of each section to provide training to student pharmacists and newly appointed junior pharmacists in their section. Thus, maintaining the future manpower requirement of hospital pharmacist.

QUESTIONS

1. Define a hospital pharmacy.

2. Write briefly about the origin and development of hospital pharmacy.

3. Write a note on the responsibilities of a hospital pharmacist.

4. Enumerate the organizational structure of a modern hospital pharmacy.

5. Explain the functions of various sections of a hospital pharmacy.

6. Describe the work of a hospital pharmacy, highlighting the qualification of the people appointed to carry out those jobs.

7. What duties are expected of a pharmacist after dispensing in a modern hospital pharmacy set up?

8. Explain the staff requirement and infrastructure of a modern hospital pharmacy.

ADVERSE DRUG REACTIONS

LEARNING OBJECTIVE

The chapter aims at providing some broad understanding of adverse drug reactions starting from its reasons, prevention, types, detection, and management. The same objectives are explained separately for drug interactions also. Some popular examples for the later are given at the end, for the students to remember while in professional practice.

INTRODUCTION

Due to a number of reasons, drugs may produce unwanted reactions in patients. These effects occur at the normal accepted dose and not at the excessive dose. Hence, there is a requirement of a careful monitoring of the patients who are under longtime therapy. Some drugs' Adverse Drug Reactions (ADR) are documented and hence known to the treating physicians. Nevertheless, they are also counted as ADR. Some other reactions which occur due to accidental overdose, prescribing or dispensing error, or intentional overdose are not included in Adverse Drug Reactions. Thus ADR can be defined as the reaction that is harmful, unintended, and occurs at doses normally used in humans for prevention, diagnosis or treatment of diseases.

Reasons or Predisposing Factors for ADR

1. **Stopping in Mid-way:** Patients often stop taking medicines due to various reasons like cost, ignorance, non-availability, etc. There is a possibility of ADR if drugs like steroids and hormones are suddenly withdrawn.

2. Factors like age, idiosyncrasy, and disease conditions also cause unwanted reactions in some patients.

3. **Bioavailability Problems:** Due to the poor formulation of drugs, blood concentration is affected and hence they may reach a toxic level in some patients, subsequently leading to ADR.

4. Intake of drugs should be stopped at an appropriate time. It should not be continued indefinitely unless otherwise indicated. Failure to set therapeutic endpoint is one of the reasons for ADR to occur. Intake of drugs like digitalis, diuretics, steroids, and antibiotics should be stopped when their continuation is not necessary.

5. Self-medication by patients and over prescription by doctors may also produce ADR. If any mishap or disease arises under a doctor's treatment, it is known as Iatrogenic or a Drug-Induced Disease.

6. **Sex:** It is a general perception that women are more susceptible to ADR than men. Though the reason is not established yet, it is suspected that it could be owed to hormonal, pharmacokinetic or immunological factor. One known example to justify this argument is the adverse effect of Chloramphenicol [Blood Dyscrasias] which is more common in the female population.

7. **Age:** The chances of drugs producing ADR on infants, young children as well as on elderly people are more due to underdevelopment of internal organs in the farmer and improper functioning of them in the later. Chloramphenicol produces 'gray baby syndrome' on the neonates whereas nitrates and ACE inhibitors cause hypotension in geriatric cases.

8. Apart from above, drug interactions is one of the major reasons for ADR

Reducing or Preventing ADR

Though Adverse Drug Reactions cannot be eliminated, they can be reduced if the drugs are used with caution and by following certain safety aspects as listed below.

1. Patient medication history should be taken into consideration before prescribing drugs.
2. Drugs should be administered only when required. If the indication is lacking, avoid using those drugs.
3. Drugs should be prescribed in the minimum possible quantity. Polypharmacy or multiple drug regimens should be avoided.
4. Children and old people are susceptible to ADR. Hence, they should be monitored during therapy.
5. Continuous review of the drug requirement should be undertaken. Based on that, the dose should be reduced or altogether stopped at an appropriate time.

Classification of ADR

Adverse Drug Reactions are classified into two different types:

- Predictable and dose-dependent
- Unpredictable and independent of dose

Type I: Predictable and dose-dependent

This type of ADRs are more common, owing to the pharmacological activities of the drug. And based on that, it can be further classified into three categories:

A. Excess pharmacological effect or toxic effect

B. Secondary pharmacological effect or side effect and

C. Return effect on stopping the drug

Type II: Unpredictable and independent of dose

This type of ADR is not very common. It only occurs in some patients due to their peculiarity. It has nothing to do with drugs' pharmacological action. At the same time, it is far more dangerous and requires immediate stopping of the drug concerned. This type can be further classified into three categories.

A. Idiosyncrasy

B. Allergy including anaphylaxis and

C. Genetic related

I A. Excess pharmacological effect or Toxic Effects: These may occur due to the excess activity of a drug caused by long-time use or drug overdose. The term drug overdose is relative. Drugs are usually given in a range of doses. Sometimes, the upper range of the permitted dose is prescribed to the patient which may result in a toxic effect in some patients. Other times, IN cases of kidney failure, liver diseases, and anemia, some drugs cause excessive pharmacological effect even in normal doses. Gentamicin in the case of kidney failure and paracetamol in liver diseases are some of the examples for cases like these. Toxic effects of almost all the drugs are documented for ready reference and monitoring. Some are given below:

1. Heparin induces bleeding

2. Streptomycin causes deafness

3. Emetine causes myocardial damage

4. Coma by barbiturates

5. Digoxin causes atrioventricular block and

6. Corticosteroids and anti-inflammatory drugs suppress the response to injury and infections.

I B. Secondary pharmacological effect or side effect: Drugs may have more functionalities even though they are prescribed for their primary activity only. Their secondary effects are nullified by either prescribing corrective drugs or formulation techniques. However, some side effects cannot be corrected using an external agent. For example, steroids weaken the defense mechanism of the patient, hence latent diseases like tuberculosis get activated. Sedation by antihistamines is another common example of secondary pharmacological side effects.

I C. Rebound Effects: Adverse effects are not only observed for the drugs which cause dependence but also for other drugs when they are stopped suddenly. Usually, the diseases for which they were used, relapse. For instance, if an antiepileptic drug is stopped suddenly, seizures may increase in those patients. Similarly, if the β.blockers are stopped, angina pectoris worsen, and hypertension results if clonidine (a hypotensive agent) is discontinued.

Another example is the stopping of addiction-forming, CNS depressants which result in tachycardia, confusion, delirium, agitation, and convulsions. These are termed as rebound response upon discontinuation of therapy. These drugs should be stopped gradually and not abruptly. Furthermore, they should be replaced with appropriate alternative drugs to prevent ADR.

II A. Idiosyncrasy: It is defined as a reaction due to certain unexpected effects of drugs because of the peculiarities of an individual. It is an unusual individual response to certain drugs by the patient. The response is unexpected, unpredictable and does not depend on the dose. For example, cinchona alkaloids like quinine and quinidine produce cramps, diarrhea, and vascular collapse in some patients. Barbiturates, instead of inducing depression, leads to excitement and mental confusion in some individuals.

II B. Allergy: This is also called drug hypersensitivity. It is important to note that not all patients experience allergic reactions to the drug. Only a small percentage of the population goes through these reactions. Contrary to popular belief, there is no sudden development. It requires prior sensitization of at least 7 to 10 days to produce the effect after first exposure. Also, the drug could become tolerable at a later stage and those who tolerated it earlier may develop allergic reactions over time. Different types of allergic reactions are produced in different individuals for the same drug and sometimes a completely different drug may produce the same type of reactions. As already pointed out, they are unpredictable and not related to dose because sometimes an increase in dose cannot produce the same reactions in other individuals.

On the other hand, anaphylaxis is an allergic reaction that is severe and sudden which may lead to loss of consciousness or even death. Photosensitivity is another type of allergic reaction exhibited by some individuals.

II. C. Genetics: Genotype of a particular individual can cause variation in the effects of drugs, hence there are possibilities for ADR. Sometimes, to produce the same effect, an increase of 500% in dose may be required for some individuals, depending on their genetics. It is because their rate of metabolism differs and we know that the rate of metabolism depends on microsomal enzymes which, in turn, is controlled by genes. The site of action and its sensitivity to drugs also play an important role in the drug's effect which differs due to genotypes.

For example, glucose 6 phosphate dehydrogenase deficiency may lead to hemolysis with Primaquine. The drugs are acetylated in the liver during metabolism if it is slow in some individuals due to genotype, there is the possibility of adverse reactions to drugs like procainamide, isoniazid, etc.

Differences between Type I and Type II ADR

No.	Type I	Type II
1	Can be predicted	Cannot be predicted
2.	Dose-related	Occurs independent of dose
3.	Commonly occurring	It is rare
4.	Not serious, very rarely cause death	It is serious and may be fatal
5.	If the dose of the drug concerned is reduced, the problem is solved.	Requires complete stopping of the drug
6.	Generally identified even before the first time marketing of the drug	Occur rarely hence require continuous post-marketing surveillance
7.	The effects of this type of ADR are qualitatively normal but quantitatively excess	The effects are unusual unexpected and harmful.

Methods of Detecting and Monitoring ADR

As it is difficult to differentiate between the disease manifestations and the Adverse Drug Reactions, the following methods are developed to identify ADR.

1. Case-control studies
2. Cohort studies
3. Spontaneous case reports and
4. Vital statistics and record linkage studies

1. **Case-Control Study:** In this study, the group of people with the disease (cases) and the group of people without the disease (control) are compared. Here, the disease selected should be induced by the drug. Additionally, patients' medication histories are collected and compared. If the drug has indeed caused the disease, its use among the cases should be far more than the controls.

   This type of study can be conducted quickly and effectively and that too at a reasonable cost. However, it requires more scientific knowledge to conduct correctly and to interpret the data obtained after the study.

   For example, in a study of the relationship between lung cancer and cigarette smoking, it was found that the chances of the disease occurring in smokers are 10 to 11 times more than non-smokers. As the connection between the two depends on the amount of smoking and the scope of other factors is almost negligible, it is safe to conclude that the result of the study is justified.

2. **Cohort Study:** Cohort is a group of people with approximately the same age, put under similar conditions, receiving the same drug. In this study, the drug under observation is given to the group and watched for varying periods to find out the ADR. This can be for a short period, say the treatment period plus a month. The study is carried out in various places of the country and up to 2000 to 3000 patients are selected for the process. Usually, the toxic effects due to excessive pharmacological effects are detected by this method. Moreover, the delayed effects of the drug can also be detected using the same method.

In the long term study lasting for a few years, up to 20,000 patients may be observed for detecting adverse drug reactions. The relevant information is collected from the doctor, pharmacist, and even the patient, if possible. However, the problem with this method is drop-outs due to migration and some other related factors. It is an expensive and difficult method known as Post Marketing Surveillance.

3. **Spontaneous Case Reports:** If a prescriber suspects any problem with the patient because of drug usage, he reports it to medical or pharmaceutical journals or to the manufacturer of the drug. This is called a spontaneous case report. This method is used to alert other prescribers.

Nowadays, ADR reporting agencies are available like the one with the World Health Organization (WHO). Once a report is sent to them with relevant particulars, they investigate and report it to all the medical practitioners through journals, newsletters, and associations, etc. This method is relatively cheaper. However, the frequency of particular ADR, its correlation with drug and disease, etc. still have to be determined. Also, it cannot be claimed to be a complete report.

4. **Vital Statistics and Record Linkage Studies:** All the health care institutions (hospitals and clinics) and local bodies are required to maintain morbidity and mortality data. From these records, disease prevailing areas and causes of death in a particular area can be collected and analyzed.

However, this method is not often successful because of the reasons like long delay in collecting data, reliability of the data, etc. If the data is sincerely entered in records and computerized, it may be useful to collect and analyze them easily in the future.

Management of Adverse Drug Reactions – Role of Pharmacists

Irrespective of the careful treatment, ADR does happen owing to multiple factors that are beyond the control of the health care team. In those unfortunate events, the pharmacists have the following functions to manage ADR.

First of all, they should review the available literature regarding the ADR of the particular drug. Any worthwhile point found should be discussed with the physicians. Next, the pharmacist should check the patient's medication history. They should also review other factors like co-administration of other drugs, stage of the disease, etc. This should be followed by an immediate Therapeutic Drug Monitoring (TDM), if not started already. The plasma concentration of the drug in the particular patient should be analyzed and whether the reaction is dose-dependent or not can be detected. Finally, depending on the seriousness of the reaction, they can advise stopping the drug. For this, they have to analyze the risk/benefit ratio and the availability of substitute drugs.

If the pharmacy and therapeutic committee [PTC] is available in a particular hospital, the pharmacist as the secretary of PTC should inform the committee about the ADR. PTC, in turn, discusses it and advises the treating physician, what to do and how to proceed with further treatment. It monitors the recovery of the patient from ADR and ensures proper treatment thereafter. Note that the pharmacist has to implement the decisions of PTC as its secretary.

All records of adverse drug reactions should be documented properly and reported to suitable higher authorities. These tasks and model ADR reporting forms are given in Chapter No. 11, Page No. 88.

DRUG INTERACTIONS

Introduction

Though drug interactions are part of adverse drug reactions, they are studied separately because of their significance. The concurrent administration of drugs to the patient is a reality and hence the possibility of drug interactions is always there. Invariably, almost all the drugs are synthetic chemicals or chemical constituents of natural drugs, and hence the potential for drug interactions is evident. Moreover, these chemicals are administered into the body where scores of biochemical are already present. Additionally, the chemical drugs received from outside are metabolized to different chemicals inside the body. Thus, we mix up a lot of chemicals in the patient's body and if we are non-vigilant throughout the course of long treatment, harmful effects cannot be avoided.

Thus, a drug interaction is defined as a situation in which the effects of one drug are altered by prior or co-administration of another drug. It also includes drug-food interactions and drug-disease interactions.

Reasons for Drug Interactions

1. **Patients consulting multiple physicians:** The patients are in a hurry to get relief from their diseases and hence they go to several physicians and even follow up with multiple systems of treatment like Ayurveda, Siddha or Homeopathy. Because of this situation, there are chances for adverse drug interactions but usually, patients purchase drugs from neighborhood pharmacies only, and hence pharmacists can counsel such patients.

2. **Simultaneous use of OTC drugs and prescription drugs:** The patients often purchase drugs for common problems from nearby pharmacies and they continue to use the same along with prescription drugs. They may not reveal it to the physician or pharmacist directly. Hence, the questions are asked cleverly using symptoms normally treated with OTC drugs and information collected.

3. **Non-compliance:** Instructions given by doctors or pharmacists regarding the use of drugs are not correctly followed by many patients. This needs attention to avoid drug-drug interactions.

4. **Drug potency:** If potent drugs are used together, the chances of harmful effects are more. For example, if antipsychotic, antidepressant and anti parkinsonism agents with anticholinergic activity are used together, it leads to dryness of mouth and blurring of vision.

5. **Drug abuse:** Some patients abuse drugs knowingly or unknowingly and hence, the interactions chances increase.

Problems in Detecting Drug Interactions

Sometimes, the patient's disease conditions are too complicated to detect ADR. If something abnormal is detected, it is considered as disease manifestation and not as probable ADR. Other times, they are attributed to factors other than drug interaction like tolerance, irregular use of the drug, etc.

The index of suspicion of many clinicians is low as they strongly believe that their treatment will not go wrong. When the problem gets out of hand, they search for earlier reports of ADR of the drug used until then they keep questioning their own observation of symptoms of ADR.

For a number of drugs, there is no measure for an activity similar to antihypertension and hypoglycemic drugs which are measured by blood pressure and blood sugar level respectively. For example, take the case of tranquilizers and analgesics, whose effect potential is not possible to detect.

Above all, if drug interaction in a patient is reported by a physician, they will be in a challenging situation followed by severe criticism and possible legal action.

Uses of Drug Interaction Reports

If the interaction between the two drugs is known, therapeutic alternatives can be used to prevent the situation. For example, we know that anticoagulant drug Warfarin interacts with Aspirin, so it should be given with paracetamol instead of aspirin. Similarly, if tetracycline and antacids have to be given together, it can be done with a time gap. Thus, the interacting drugs are given by following adjustments like changing doses or close monitoring of therapy.

Some interactions are beneficial and are used in favor of the patients. For instance, probenecid, if given together with penicillin increases the duration of action of the later. Hence, the dose of penicillin is reduced.

All reported drug interactions need not produce the same effect in all the patients. It depends on variables like age, genetics, renal disease, hepatic disorders, drinking habit, smoking, food intake, etc. Each of these variables influences the effect of the drug, therefore drugs interactions reports should be based on the present case. Moreover, some interactions are reported based on animal studies. They need not be the same in the human body.

It was found that if a person is exposed to DDT pesticide, the metabolism of some drugs is affected. So, even the environment can affect the drug's activity, hence the need for dose or therapy adjustment becomes very clear.

Classification of Drug Interactions

Depending on the benefit and some other factors, drug interactions are classified into two types:

1. Beneficial interactions

2. Adverse interactions

1. **Beneficial interactions:** Few drugs, on interaction with other drugs produce beneficial effects. Potentiation or synergisms are some of the examples of such benefits. Some drugs are used deliberately to enhance the effect of other drugs or minimize the unwanted effect of it. The examples are sulphamethoxazole and trimethoprim combination, and carbidopa and levodopa respectively. There are many formulations in the market using these beneficial effects like the estrogen-progestogen combination as contraceptive, ampicillin, cloxacillin combination as a potent antibiotic, and β.blockers-diuretic combination as hypotensive agents.

Drug interactions can also be used to treat the patients struggling with drug overdose as they nullify or antagonize the adverse effect of overdose drug. The examples are levodopa and vitamin B6, warfarin and vitamin K, narcotic analgesics and nalorphine.

2. **Adverse interactions:** Due to the introduction of newer drugs for treatment and prescribing multiple drugs, the possibility for adverse interactions also increases day by day. These adverse reactions can be put under two broad classifications:

   1. Pharmacodynamic drug interactions

   2. Pharmacokinetic drug interactions

If the drug interactions are based on their effect on the body, they are called pharmacodynamic drug interactions and if they are due to absorption, distribution, metabolism or excretion of the drug, they are referred to as pharmacokinetic interactions.

1. Pharmacodynamic Drug Interactions

These interactions happen when two drugs with the same effects are concurrently administered unknowingly. All the beneficial interactions listed above are also based on the activity of the drugs only. Some of the adverse interactions due to drug activities are listed below:

If hypnotics are given with antihistamines, narcotic analgesics, tranquilizers or alcohol, their effect is increased drastically resulting in unwanted proportions. Hence, the combinations of CNS depressants should be avoided but sometimes it is overlooked or hidden from the prescribers.

Digoxin and quinidine combination is another example of a pharmacodynamic drug interaction. The basic properties of all the drugs prescribed should be remembered by prescribers and pharmacists to avoid such problems.

2. Pharmacokinetic Drug Interactions

These interactions are due to

1. Change in the absorption of drugs
2. Alteration in protein binding and distribution
3. Biotransformation changes and
4. Drug elimination problems

(i) **Change in the absorption of drugs:** Iron preparations and drugs containing calcium, magnesium, and aluminum (antacids) precipitate or chelate tetracyclines, hence, its absorption from the GI tract is affected. Propantheline, if administered along with digoxin or pethidine shows delays in the absorption.

(ii) **Alteration in distribution:** If chloral hydrate is given with warfarin, trichloroacetic acid, the metabolite of the former displaces the warfarin from its protein binding sites. Hence, Warfarin concentration in the blood increases to double the quantity. However, it is temporary as clearance increases correspondingly.

(iii) **Biotransformation changes:** Some drugs increase the drug-metabolizing enzymes, others decrease it. Hence, there are changes in plasma drug concentration and drug activity which either decreases or increases. If the given drug produces pharmacological activity, it is reduced by the induction of enzymes. And, if the metabolite is responsible for drug activity, it is increased. An example for this type of situation is the co-administration of phenylbutazone and phenytoin. Here, the phenytoin effect is increased by the induction of the enzyme by phenylbutazone. Similarly, when allopurinol and mercaptopurine are given together metabolizing enzymes are inhibited by Allopurinol, hence, 6 mercaptopurine metabolism is delayed and its toxic effect is increased. The dose of 6 mercaptopurine should be reduced in such cases.

(iv) **Drug elimination problems:** Some drugs, if administered together compete for elimination via active tubular secretion. As a result, each of these drugs eliminates slowly and consequently stays longer inside the body. The duration of action thus increases. One example that has already been mentioned is probenecid and penicillin, another one is salicylates and uricosuric agents.

If we alter the pH of the urine, the drug's elimination is affected. This type of drug interaction is used for treating poison cases. For example, if we make urine pH alkaline using sodium bicarbonate, acidic drugs like salicylates and phenobarbitone are eliminated quickly from the body. Similarly, if we make urine pH acidic using ammonium chloride alkaline drugs like quinidine is eliminated faster.

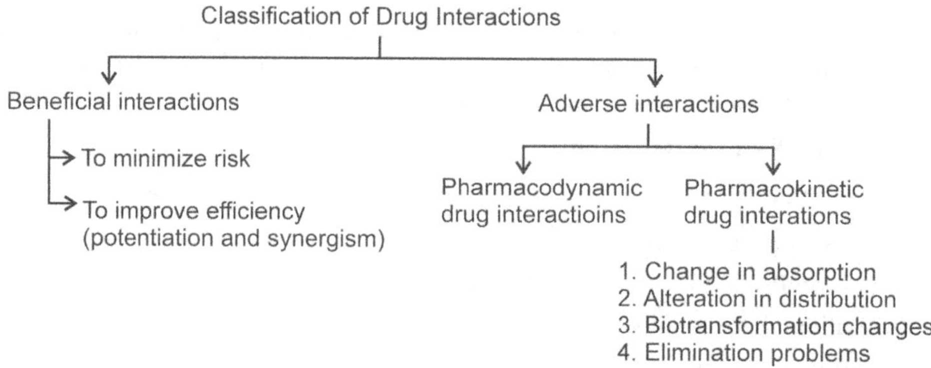

Drug Interaction Examples

I. Analgesics	
1. Aspirin with Alcohol	GI irritation and bleeding
2. Aspirin with Ibuprofen	No superior action
3. Narcotic analgesics with CNS depressants like barbiturates	Excessive depressant action
4. Paracetamol with Metoclopramide	The increased onset of Paracetamol action
II. Cardio Vascular Agents	
1. Digitalis and its preparations with barbiturates	Increase the metabolism of Digoxin hence, more dose may be required
2. Digitalis and its preparations with Diuretics	Potassium depletion, give KCl tablets. If not, heart become sensitive to Digitalis and its toxicity
3. Digitalis and its preparations with Reserpine	Increased risk of cardiac arrest
4. Methyl Dopa with Levodopa	Potentiation, so reduce dose.
5. Propranolol with Insulin, Tolbutamide etc	Increase the action of hypoglycemic agents, results in acute hypoglycemia. Additional danger is that effect is not noticeable till serious stage
6. Anticoagulants Warfarin etc with	
(a) Aspirin	Increased effect
(b) Antacids	Decreased effect
(c) Chloromphenicol	Increased effect
(d) Phenylbutazone and oxyphenbutazone	Increase anticoagulant effect
(e) Phenytoin	Phenytoin effect increases, anticoagulant effect decreases
(f) Vitamin K	Antagonism
III. GI Agents	
1. Antacids with Bisacodyl	GI irritation due to disintegration of enteric coating in stomach itself.
2. Antacids with Tetracycline	Metal ions in antacids like Ca, Mg, Al form complex with Tetracycline, so poorabsorption
IV. Hypoglycemic Agents	
Insulin, Tolbutamide, etc with 1. Corticosteroids like Prednisolone	Increase the blood glucose level
2. Alcohol	Different effects with various intake quantities, may induce faster hypoglycemia
3. Propranolol	Increase the action of insulin etc
4. Coumarin (anticoagulant)	Increase in action due to decrease in metabolism. Reduce dose.
5. Phenylbutazone	Increase the action, so reduce dose

V. Psychopharmacological Agents	
With alcohol	More CNS Depressant action. Hence avoid it.
1. Antidepressants with	
(a) Coumarin	Increase the effect of anti coagulants
(b) MAO inhibitors	Tremors, convulsions
(c) Reserpine	Contraindicated
2. Antipsychotic agents (chlorpromazine group) with	
(a) Antacids	Magnesium trisilicate decrease plasma level of the drug. Avoid or delay
(b) Anticholinergics	Dryness of mouth, blurring of vision, constipation, and urine detention
(c) Levodopa	Action of Levodopa inhibited
(d) MAO Inhibitors	Increase the action of the antipsychotic drugs
(c) Levodopa	Action of Levodopa inhibited
(d) MAO Inhibitors	Increase the action of the antipsychotic drugs
3. Sedatives and Hypnotics with	
(a) Alcohol	Enhanced CNS depression
(b) MAO inhibitors	Enhanced CNS depression so avoid it
(c) Digitoxin	Increase the rate of metabolism of Digitoxin
(d) Griseofulvin	Decrease in action of Griseofulvin
VI. Vitamins	
1. Folic acid with Phenytoin	Development of Folic acid deficiency and reduced Phenytoin level
2. Vitamin B_6 with Levodopa	Antagonism patients under Levodopa therapy should avoidmultivitamins
3. Vitamin C with Aspirin	Reduced Vitamin C absorption
4. Vitamin D with Phenytoin	Increase the metabolism of Vitamin D, so Vitamin D deficiency (Rickets, etc)
5. Vitamin K with Coumarin	Antagonism

QUESTIONS

1. Define ADR.
2. Classify ADR.
3. Discuss the reasons for ADR.
4. How can ADR be reduced?
5. List the differences between the two types of ADR.
6. Define Drug-Drug interaction and what are the two types of Drug Interactions?
7. What are the reasons for Drug-Drug Interactions?

8. What are the problems in detecting drug interactions?

9. How can we use the Drug Interaction information?

10. Explain the Type I and Type II ADRs in detail with examples.

11. Enumerate various methods of detecting or monitoring ADR.

12. How is ADR managed? Discuss the role of a pharmacist.

13. Classify drug interactions. Explain each one of them with examples.

14. What are pharmacokinetic drug interactions? Give examples.

Chapter **4**

COMMUNITY PHARMACY

LEARNING OBJECTIVE

The objective of the chapter is to provide comprehensive knowledge about community pharmacy which many students wish to start after the completion of the course. Its organization, types and design and more importantly its legal requirements are explained in detail. Records to be maintained are mentioned at the end of the chapter. They are all given both for retail and wholesale trade in medicine.

As the name indicates, a community pharmacy is an organization functioning in the midst of a community of an area and provides drugs and other health services to the people. According to James W. Richards, *"community pharmacy is defined as an establishment, that is privately owned and whose functions in varying degrees, is to serve society's need for both drug products and pharmaceutical services."* It is generally recognized by the public as the most accessible source of drugs and drug information.

The community pharmacies in India are still old fashioned, mostly product-oriented and functioning with a commercial background. On the other hand, developed countries have modern community pharmacies that are patient-oriented and providing pharmaceutical care to the people. This is because those pharmacies have highly qualified (M.Pharm. or Pharm.D) pharmacists, unlike D.Pharm pharmacists we have in India. It is high time for moving on to new roles, new responsibilities, and accountability as per senior pharmacists and well-wishers of the pharmacy profession.

ORGANIZATION

While organizing a community pharmacy, the very first thing one must consider is its location. Hence, the site selection for the pharmacy assumes more importance. Needless to mention, the best site for a pharmacy is the place where most patients visit nearby practicing physicians. So, it should be established in a place close to the clinics of practicing physicians. As the viability of a community pharmacy largely depends on the prescription flow, it must be located where more physicians practice. It could also be close to hospitals where a large number of patients visit.

The next best site could be near the heart of the village, town or a city where a lot of people go shopping and the floating population is more. Here, the people bring the prescription for purchase, old prescriptions for refilling or for OTC medicines even from far off places. Thus, the survival of a pharmacy established here is guaranteed and success is almost certain. However, the problem with the site is the accumulation of a large number of competing pharmacies and thereby cutting into each other's business. Hence, the supply should be proportionate to the demand. As per the rules set up by some governments, there should be some minimum distance between two pharmacies to avoid overcrowding in one area and leaving other areas without any pharmacy. Thereby, they also ensure that drug availability spread evenly across the community.

The third viable site to establish a pharmacy is in a newly developed area or the colonies of cities where a considerable number of people live. People always tend to purchase from neighborhood pharmacies to ensure, regular, immediate and uninterrupted supply of medicines. Hence, establishing contact with local people is important for a community pharmacist. As the area of residence grows and spreads, the community pharmacy gets the advantage of a prior set up. Here, the growth is rather slow but steady.

Apart from the above three sites, pharmacies can be established inside Bus Stands, Railway Stations, Shopping malls, and even in large apartment complexes. Each of these places has its own merits and demerits. Nevertheless, they offer a choice if other locations are ruled out.

Structure

The structure and organization of a community pharmacy can take three forms. Both retail and wholesale pharmacies fall under these three categories. They are:

1. Sole Proprietary concerns

2. Partnership concerns

3. Corporations.

1. Sole Proprietary Concerns

These are small and less complex organization and the majority of community pharmacies fall under this type. They are established by an individual with their own or borrowed capital, hence, the risks involved in the business, as well as the profit, concern only one individual. Being the sole owner of the pharmacy, they can decide the manner of conducting business but it should be within the framework of the law. In this type of pharmacies, the proprietor uses their personal assets to meet the obligations of the business and vice versa i.e. business assets may be used to satisfy their personal commitments. They can develop and expand the organization or wrap up whenever they want.

2. Partnership Concerns

These establishments are formed by two or more individuals based on some contract or a deed. This deed is for the smooth functioning of the organization and to prevent any future disagreement. As per the agreement, tasks, profit or loss, and management of the firm are divided among the partners. Usually, partnership firms are formed when the resources of an individual are not sufficient. Otherwise, it is almost like sole proprietorship concern that does not require government permission to establish or to dissolve.

3. Corporations

These have to be established by government permission as they are legal entities. They are created with the share capital collected from the general public and that is why they require government nod and some control. The shareholders have limited liability to the extent of their share in the business. As it is not dependent on any individual, death or nonfunctioning of a shareholder or transfer of shares from one individual to another will not affect the existence of the organization. However, establishing these corporations is a complex process. They cannot be dissolved as per the wish of the shareholder; instead, they require government permission. An example of this type of pharmacies is the chain of pharmacies sharing the same name.

Types and Design

There are three types of community pharmacies depending on the size and services they provide to the customers. They are 1. Small scale ordinary type 2. Large scale superstore type 3. Modern patient-oriented type.

1. Small scale ordinary type

It is established in a minimum floor area required by the law, usually around 120 sq.feet. A large portion of it is allotted for the display of drugs and remaining for a sales and dispensing counter. For cold storage, a refrigerator is available but a large number of goods cannot be stored here. Except for dispensing to the customer, no other patient service is provided in this type of pharmacy. The limited stock of other general items like cosmetics, baby food, etc is also sold here. There may be two or three employees depending upon the business volume. It is more or less like a general store in the area. Limited working hours, limited stock and limited space are the disadvantages of this type of pharmacy. However, it satisfies the basic needs of a community by providing common drugs across the counter.

2. Large scale superstore type

It is established in a big floor area, say about 500 sq.ft. It has a large display area and customer movement area inside the pharmacy. Items like cosmetics and other general utilities may be displayed outside the sales counter in the customer area for self picking by the customers. Except for the availability of huge and variety of goods, it is not that different from the former type. Here, except for dispensing, no other professional service is provided. However, a lot of stock and extended working hours are their advantage which is an attracting factor for customers as they are assured of the availability of all items and drugs in a big store like this. Customers usually prefer purchasing all that they require at one shop. Big overhead expenses, the large amount of capital requirement, loss due to less patronage are some of the disadvantages of this type of pharmacies.

3. Modern patient-oriented type

Modern community pharmacies are the ones that have room for patient-oriented services. These pharmacies engage highly qualified pharmacists with M.Pharm or Pharm.D degree and relevant experience in the field. Apart from the usual area for display and dispensing of drugs, these pharmacies provide a place for patient counseling and consultation. Their doubts about drug usage, its side effects, personal bodily problems, etc are discussed here in privacy. Simple tests like monitoring blood pressure, blood sugar are also conducted here.

The patient consultation area is nothing but a small clinic where physicians are available for a few hours in a day to consult patients. Simply put, it is a clinic inside a pharmacy as opposed to the usual pharmacy inside a clinic. These services are available in modern pharmacies of developed countries. Various specialists like skin, dental, pediatric and gynecologists are available for few fixed hours on fixed days in these pharmacies, thus offering a great service to pharmacy customers. The services available in our neighborhood, that too in easily approachable pharmacies go a long way in disease prevention, spreading and treatment before it gets complicated due to delay in getting medical attention which is often the case with many of us. Needless to mention, these pharmacies have large patient movement area with facilities for selecting and picking general and cosmetic products from among a large number of brands and manufacturers. These pharmacies project a completely professional atmosphere unlike our Indian pharmacies with the commercial look.

Layout and Design

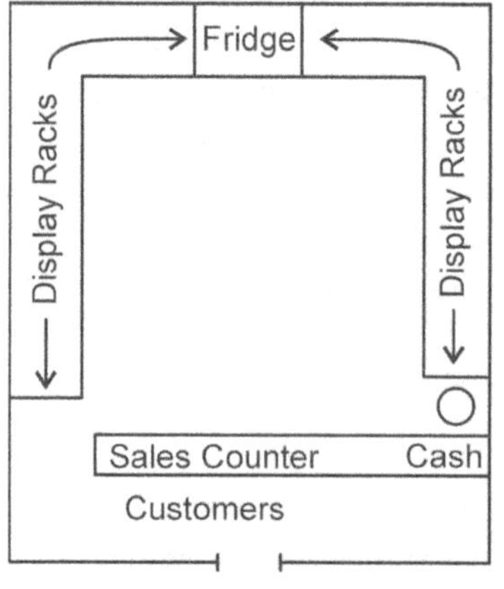

Layout of Small Scale Pharmacy

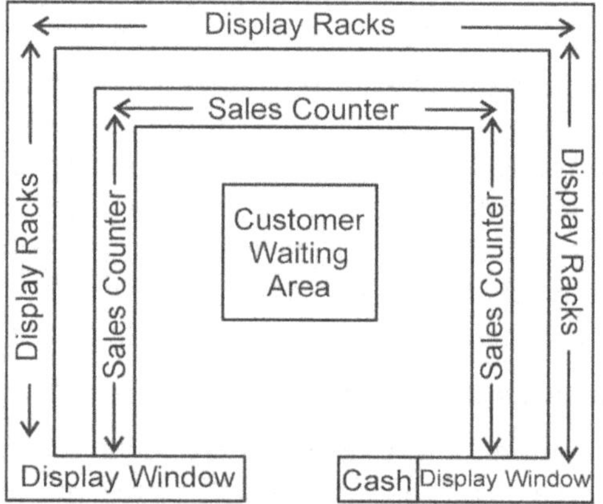

Layout of Medium Scale Pharmacy

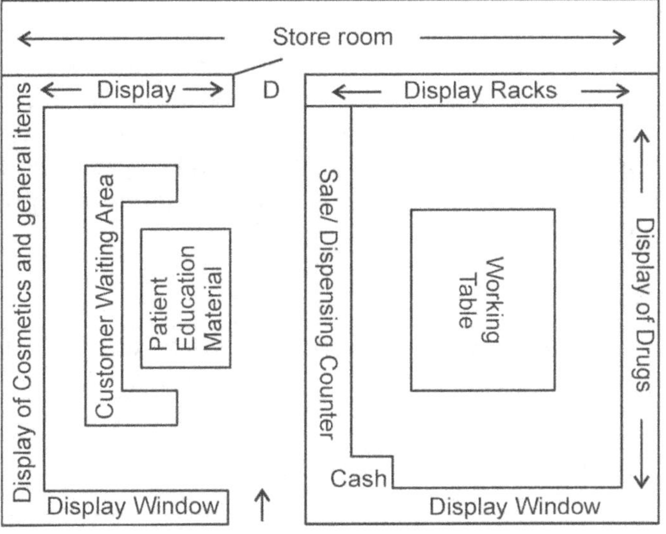

Layout of Large Scale Pharmacy

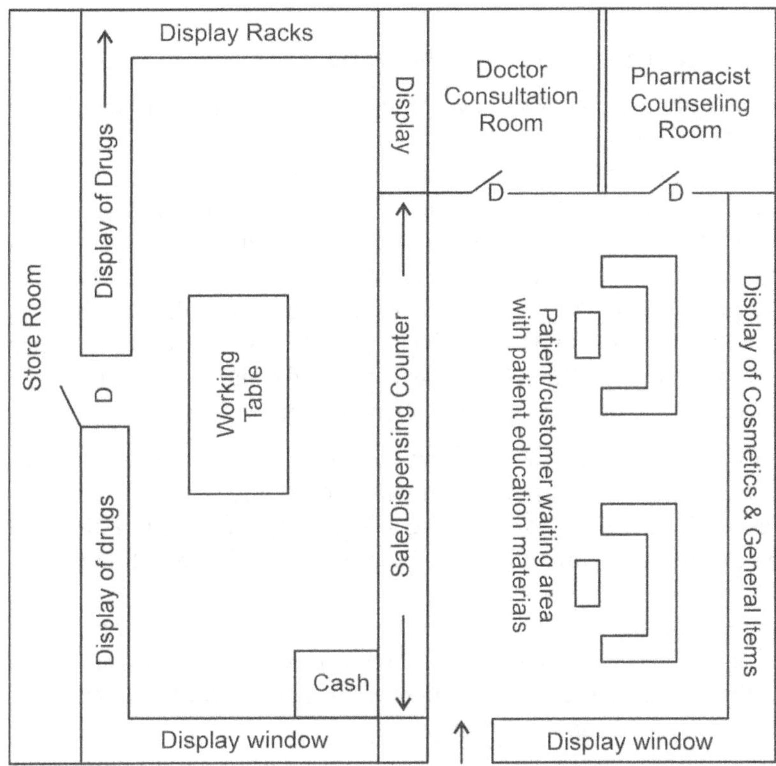

Layout of Modern Patient Oriented Retail Pharmacy

Legal Requirement

For starting a wholesale or retail pharmacy, a license from the drug control department is required. The procedure to obtain a license is given in detail in the Drugs and Cosmetics Act and rules. Students are advised to go through it for detail. Separate licenses are issued for schedule C and C1 drugs, those other than in schedule C and C1, and also for schedule X drugs (both retail and whole trade). These licenses require specific forms to apply, renew and receive. They are given in the table below:

Licenses and Forms

License FOR	DRUGS OTHER THAN SCH.C AND C1	DRUGS IN SCH. C AND C1	DRUGS IN SCH.X
RETAIL	20	21	20F
RESTRICTED LICENCE	20A	21A	---
WHOLESALE	20B	21B	20G
WHOLESALE FROM MOTOR VEHICLE	20BB	21BB	----

The Legal Requirement for starting Wholesale

Strangely in India, a pharmacist was not required for starting the wholesale in drugs until recently. Now, the Government of India has brought in amendments to the D and C act and thereby a pharmacist has to be appointed for setting up wholesale. However, this amendment is yet to be implemented owing to the backlash from wholesale traders. As of now, matriculates with 3 years experience or any graduate with one year experience in the drug trade are eligible for starting a wholesale trade in medicine. That apart, 10 sq.Mt floor area, facilities for proper storage are also required to set it up. The wholesale traders should sell the drugs only to retail license holders, however, hospitals, institutions, officers authorized to purchase for the government are exempted from this rule. The records for purchase, sale, and stock should be maintained and shown to the drugs inspector during the inspection.

The wholesale traders are otherwise known as stockists of one or more companies where only the products of those companies are available. Some stockists are given the right to promote the sale of drugs of a particular company by propaganda for which they get a physician's sample, propaganda materials, and credits from the manufacturers. They are called Propaganda cum Distributors. They appoint sales representatives to take orders from hospitals and retail pharmacies and have delivery boys and vehicles for the same. Another form of the wholesale is from the regional depots of manufacturers who establish such depots in important big cities and thereby reducing marketing expenses by saving wholesale traders commission and vendor's lead time (time taken for supply of goods).

The Legal Requirement for Starting the Retail Sale

There are 3 types of licenses issued for retail trade. They are:

1. Drugs store

2. Chemists and Druggists

3. Pharmacy

1. **Drug store:** The licenses issued for these stores are known as restricted licenses because the licensee cannot sell all the drugs but only those permitted by the license. These stores sell the usual household remedies and medicines only as they are not accompanied by the services of a qualified pharmacist. The licensee should store the drugs properly in order to preserve their potency.

2. **Chemists and druggists:** These are the pharmacies we commonly call medical shops or stores. They have full-time pharmacists for dispensing medicine. Area-wise, they require about 120 sq ft of space and proper storage facilities for these outlets. They should maintain the purchase, sale and stock register separately for schedule C and C1 drugs and schedule X drugs. They must also be equipped with refrigerators and air conditioners.

3. **Pharmacy:** A pharmacy, according to the D and C act is a place where apart from usual dispensing of pre-packed drugs, some drugs are compounded and prepared by a registered pharmacist as per prescription. Hence, they should have the required apparatus, a proper place, and facilities for the same. Just like dispensing (pharmaceutics) lab of a pharmacy institution, they should also have dispensing balance, table, tile, spatula, mortar and pestle, measuring cylinders and other glassware. These requirements are listed in Schedule N of the Drugs and Cosmetics Rules. Any person who intends to start the pharmacy must follow these rules. It is important that only registered pharmacist compounds and prepares the drugs as mentioned in the prescription. They should record those details in a separate register and account it. During the old days, pharmacies used to carry out these activities but now they have stopped.

Apart from the above 3 types of retail trades, the government is also giving a license to sell drugs from vehicles with some restrictions. For example, they are not permitted to sell schedule X drugs through these mobile pharmacies and they should also maintain proper storage conditions for the drugs.

Dispensing of Proprietary Products

Proprietary products are "Drugs or products presented in a form ready for internal or external administration of human beings or animals that are not included in the edition of Indian Pharmacopoeia for the time being or any other pharmacopeia authorized by the central govt after consultation with Drugs Technical Advisory Board"

Proprietary products are the proprietary of the company which manufactures it as per its own formula and method of manufacture after approval from the drugs controller. The formula may be patented and disclosed to the Drugs control department and there cannot be any secret ingredient in it. The manufacturer gives the products brand names to promote them among health care professionals for marketing and proper use by the proprietor of the brand. These products are dispensed by two methods. They are,

1. From the manufacturer's bulk container

This includes,

A) Measuring the required volume of the liquid drug from bulk containers supplied by the manufacturer and dispensing to patients after proper labeling.

B) Counting the number of unit dosage forms like a tablet or capsules from the bulk supply and dispensing in a proper container with the required label.

There are few exemptions for the above procedure that some proprietary preparations require addition of vehicle [water] during dispensing.

2. Dispensing manufacturers original pack

Often, manufacturers themselves market medicines in prescribed quantities and hence they can be dispensed in their original packaging. However, any literature or packing inserts with the original packaging should be removed if it is not for patients. Furthermore, any extra information that the patients need to know can be affixed on the pack of the dispensing labels without concealing the printed matter on the original label. Examples for the above type of packing are aerosol and ointments.

Maintenance of Records of Retail and Wholesale Drug Stores

There are three types of records maintained by drug traders out of which the first two are common for both retail and wholesale trades and the third one is for the retail pharmacy only. They are,

1. Legal records
2. Financial records
3. Patient records

1. **Legal records:** These are the records both retail and wholesale traders should maintain as per the D and C act and rules. They are,

   1) purchase records
   2) stock register
   3) sales register
   4) separate schedule drugs sales register
   5) schedule X sales register
   6) prescription file for schedule X drugs
   7) inspection register
   8) communication file (official letters and circulars from drug control and other government departments). Some records like prescription file for schedule X drugs are not required for wholesale trade.

2. **Financial records:** These are the records that are required to run the pharmacy efficiently and to satisfy the tax obligation. They are discussed in detail in the chapter on inventory control and drug store business management.

The records required are,

1) daybook

2) journal

3) ledger

4) profit and loss account including trial balance and balance sheet.

5) Tax notices, Receipts and other particulars file (income tax, GST, etc)

6) Insurance file

7) Salary register

8) miscellaneous file (Rent, Electric bill, Telephone bill, etc)

9) Employees' salary, service, and leave register. Financial records include Purchase, Sale, and Stock Registers. As they are shown above as legal records not repeated here.

3. **Patient records:** These are maintained by a few pharmacies only. The modern pharmacies offering patient-oriented services earn name, fame, and goodwill and thereby money from these value-added services.

The records are,

1) Patient medication profile (History)

2) Patient's family members medication profile and

3) Copies of important prescriptions, Lab reports, etc of selected patients for future reference, guidance, and counseling.

All the above records are maintained as hard copies wherever necessary and also as soft copies in pharmacy computers with facilities for easy retrieval. The government has permitted an electronic form of bookkeeping (e.files) considering the enormous and complex work involved in the process. Hence, a pharmacist must pay due attention to this work and should also learn the art and science of record keeping.

QUESTIONS

1. Write a note on Structure of a community Pharmacy

2. What are the various types and designs of a community Pharmacy?

3. How will you dispense proprietary products?

4. Describe the legal requirement for starting wholesale

5. Explain the legal requirement for starting retail sale

6. Write about the maintenance of records of retail and wholesale drug stores

CHAPTER 5

DRUGS DISTRIBUTION SYSTEM IN A HOSPITAL

LEARNING OBJECTIVE

On completion of the chapter, the student should able to explain the various systems followed in different hospitals for the distribution of drugs to both inpatients and outpatients. The principles behind pricing and charging of drugs supplied to the patient should also be remembered. More importantly, he should able to follow the legal requirements of dispensing Narcotics and Psychotropic drugs to the patient.

INTRODUCTION

The drug distribution system in hospitals can be broadly classified into two types. They are,

1. Distribution to outpatients or ambulatory patients.

2. Distribution to inpatients or institutionalized patients.

An outpatient or ambulatory patient is the one who receives treatment after consultation and diagnosis, without having to get admitted to the hospital. On the other hand, a patient who requires hospitalization for any kind of treatment is known as an inpatient. Generally, the diseases concerning outpatients are of the nature that does not require more than a few days of treatment. However, there are some exceptions like diabetes, TB and, asthma. The inpatient's problems are more complex and serious and may require close supervision, observation, and treatment for a comparatively long time. Hence, these categories of patients are admitted to the wards.

Distribution to Outpatients

As the distribution of drugs to outpatients is not complex compared to inpatients, all the type of hospitals follow the same system. After consultation and diagnosis, patients are given their prescriptions along with small chits [token] mentioning hospital numbers, names of the medicines prescribed and the quantity, as suggested by the doctors. Then the patients or their helpers take the prescription to the dispensary/pharmacy situated near the main entrance of the hospital to collect medicine which is usually the final task before moving out of the hospital.

The drugs are issued to the patients through multiple counters in the pharmacy for male and female patients. Depending on the crowd or number of outpatients coming to the hospitals, the authorities may open more counters.

At least one, if required, more pharmacists will receive prescriptions through these counters and dispense the medicines. The outpatients receive their medicines on the prescriptions given to them by the doctors of that particular hospital only. The medicines are supplied either free of cost (as in government hospitals) or on making the payment (as in private hospitals). Free medicine can be directly obtained from the pharmacy. While for paid medicines, the transaction is done at the cash counter of the hospital or by the dispensing pharmacist himself to generate the receipt. The patient can produce the receipt along with the prescription at the pharmacy to get the medicines.

Drugs are then dispensed to the patients or their helpers along with the necessary instructions regarding their use, storage, etc. These are mentioned orally as well as in written form on the containers or envelops of the medicine. The prescription or the small piece of paper (token) is retained by the pharmacist. They file the retained prescription or 'token' after writing accounts for the mentioned drugs along with the patient's hospital registration number and date. If the case sheets and prescriptions are retained, they are sent back to the hospital patient registration counter, after accounting. The patients can get them on their subsequent visits to the hospital.

Usually, seating arrangements are made for the outpatients to sit during the waiting period to get the drugs. Additionally, similar dispensing counters are opened at multiple places inside the hospital, depending upon the requirement or policy of the hospital. Sometimes, special counters are opened to dispense to the special category of patients like Non gazetted Government officers (NGGO).

Dispensing to Inpatients

There are four systems for distributing or dispensing drugs to inpatients. They are,

1. Individual prescription order system.

2. Complete floor stock system.

3. Combination of the above two systems.

4. Unit dose distribution system.

1. Individual prescription order system

This system is generally followed in small and private hospitals where wards for a larger number of patients are not available. As the name implies, the patients are given prescriptions individually, since there may be a demand for personalized service. In these small hospitals, a number of small rooms form the inpatient area with 2 to 4 beds in each room. Sometimes, individual rooms are also provided to the patients. Hence, the bulk stock of drugs in the wards (as followed in the next type of system) is not feasible here. The patients receive drugs either from the pharmacy of the hospital or purchase it from outside the pharmacy. The duty nurse administers the drug as directed in the prescription or case sheet. The advantages of this system are

1. Prescription is dispensed by the pharmacist.
2. As drugs are not stored in this inpatient area, there is closer control over the inventory by a pharmacist.
3. The patient can interact with all the members of the health care team, viz, the doctor, nurse, and pharmacist.

The main disadvantage of this type of system is the possible delay in getting the required drugs by the patients and increased cost.

2.   Complete floor stock system

In this system, medicines are brought from the main pharmacy and stored in a cupboard in each ward/floor of the hospital complex. The nurse of the ward is in charge of these medicines. They distribute the drugs to the inpatients and maintain their accounts. Under this system, the nursing station carries both 'charge' and 'non-charge' patient medications. The rarely used expensive medicines are omitted from floor stock but are dispensed upon receipt of a prescription for any individual patients. The selection of drugs to be stored in each floor/ward is done by the PTC of the hospital. In short, this is a mini pharmacy inside the ward – a ward pharmacy, but without a pharmacist. This system is used most often in government and other hospitals in which charges are not collected from the patient, or when the 'all inclusive' rate is used for charging. The following are the advantages and disadvantages of this system.

Advantages

1. Drugs are readily available in the ward.
2. There is no need to return the drugs to pharmacy or stores.
3. The pharmacy workload is reduced.
4. Consequently, the number of pharmacists required is also reduced.

Disadvantages

1. Pharmacist's services are eliminated (since dispensing is done by nurses).
2. The workload of nurses increases.
3. There are greater chances for pilferage of drugs as they are stored in dozens of wards.
4. For the same reason, more drugs need to be purchased and consequently cost to the hospital increases.
5. The medication error may increase as there is no review of prescriptions by the pharmacists.

6. Proper storage facilities need to be offered in each ward necessitating capital expenses. If not provided, drugs may deteriorate and become dangerous to patients.

3.   Combination of system 1 and 2

In some hospitals, the combination of the above two systems is followed. The individual prescription order system being the main means of distributing drugs to the patients and also limiting the use of floor stock. This combination system is probably the most commonly used system in medium and large hospitals where there is a significant number of small rooms for patients. These are known as special wards while the big halls are referred to as general wards.

4.   Unit dose distribution system

"Unit dose medications are those which are ordered, packed, handled, administered, and charged in multiples of single-dose units containing a predetermined amount of drug or supply sufficient for one regular dose, application or use". If drugs are supplied in bulk packing, unit doses are deemed necessary for dispensing to the inpatients by the nurses as they are required to make calculations, measure, weigh, and pack to administer some drugs to the inpatients. In order to avoid this unnecessary workload to the nurses, a unit dose system was introduced. It should not be confused with what we now call as the unit dose. In the above system, medicines are not to be sent to the wards in bulk containers, instead, they are subdivided, prepacked for a dose and labeled. Then, as per the request of ward nurses, they are sent in the required number of unit doses to the ward.

With the introduction and widespread use of tablets and capsules, these tasks for the pharmacists are highly minimized. The tablets and capsules are the best ready to use, unit dose forms, available in strips or blister packing. Nevertheless, few drugs like powders and cough syrups are still supplied to the hospitals in bulk containers.

The unit dose system under discussion can be best understood by the following example.

Consider an inpatient who has been prescribed a cough syrup. If only 5 L jars or 500 ml bottle packing of cough syrup is supplied to the hospital, the pharmacist has no option but to send one full container to the ward. Then, the nurses need to measure the dose every time and give it to the patient from the bulk container and keep the balance quantity within the ward.

"How to account this supply in stores or dispensary" is a major problem here. The quantity supplied can neither be debited in one patient's account nor can it be unaccounted until all the supply is consumed. Hence, there is a compulsion to go for unit dose system or smaller packing which requires empty containers, workspace, equipment for filling, sealing, labeling, etc in the dispensary.

Nowadays, this problem is solved by requesting the drug supplier to the hospital or hospital manufacturing unit to supply both bulk packing (for outpatient dispensing) and unit dose or small packing (for inpatients). However, as "distribution of drugs to the inpatients by nurses" is still followed in the majority of the hospitals, it is important to study the advantages and disadvantages of the unit dose system.

Advantages

1. The workload for nurses is reduced.

2. Wastage of drugs is reduced as the unused unit doses can be returned to the pharmacy and need not be discarded as in bulk packing.

3. Maintenance of records is made easy as this is done in multiplies of unit doses.

4. Accurate delivery of medication (in the form of unit doses) is ensured due to stringent repacking conditions and expert handling (pharmacist).

5. Above all, the unit doses are supplied with proper labels indicating the name of the medicine, its strength, quantity, and expiry date, etc., thereby wrong administration can be minimized.

Disadvantages

1. The cost of medicines goes up due to smaller packing or repacking.

2. Require more space for storage.

3. Capital expenses need to be made to establish a repacking unit in the hospital if the drugs are not supplied in unit doses.

4. The root cause for the problem is the distribution of drugs to the inpatients by nurses [not by pharmacists].

Other Systems of Dispensing to Inpatients

As discussed above, the main disadvantage of the above systems is dispensing by non-pharmacists. The pharmacists are being deprived of their tasks and hence their expertise, experience, and service cannot be used in dispensing. This leads to several problems that have already been pointed out as disadvantages of these systems. In order to overcome this problem, some hospitals have introduced a system in which the inpatient prescription or its copy is sent to the main dispensary where the pharmacist review the prescription and dispense the medicines as follows:

1. Basket (or) envelopes method

In this method, the prescribed drugs for a particular patient is put in a basket or envelope with its methods of use and other details and sent to the ward concerned. There, the nurse administers the drug to the particular patient and conveys the directions as mentioned by the pharmacist on the envelope or on a piece of paper kept inside the basket. The next day, the same basket or envelope is returned to the dispensary for further dispensing of the drugs.

Thus, the main disadvantage of not handling of prescription by the pharmacist is solved in this method. The pharmacist is able to find out incompatibility, drug interaction possibilities, and other connected problems by handling the prescription. They are able to help the doctor in selecting suitable drug/formulation for the particular patient. However, there is one loophole in this method which is the lack of pharmacist-patient direct dialogue. The communication here is carried out via a third party- the nurses.

Thus, the basket or envelop system does not solve all the problems of inpatient dispensing.

2. Mobile dispensing system

It utilizes a specially constructed stainless steel truck in which essential and frequently used medicines are taken to the wards. A worker of the pharmacy department pushes this truck to the ward accompanied by a pharmacist. It is stopped in front of each ward or at specified places and the pharmacist dispenses to the inpatients by collecting their prescriptions individually from them. The process is similar to the distribution of food and diet to the inpatients by hospital authorities, three times a day, supervised by the dieticians of the hospital. The frequency of the delivery of medicines and the hours during which the mobile unit visits the ward is selected in cooperation with the nursing service.

The main advantage of this system is that the pharmacists can dispense themselves and hence, their services are available for consultation by patients, nurses, and medical staff. However, the disadvantage of this method is the non-availability of all medicines in the truck as well as space for keeping the required quantity. So, the pharmacist or their assistants are compelled to return to the dispensary more often to bring and supply unavailable items to the inpatients. Although the two main problems associated with the previous methods- prescription handling and conveying instructions directly to the inpatients are solved, a new problem of inadequate availability of drugs arises in this method.

3. Satellite pharmacy

These are nothing but the branches of the main hospital pharmacy functioning around the hospital in a different block if the hospital is spread over a vast area on multiple floors of a building or several different buildings. The main pharmacy will supply the medicines to these satellite or mini pharmacies. The patients and the nurses in charge of the ward obtain their requirements of drugs from these satellite pharmacies instead of going to the main pharmacy. Sometimes, these satellite pharmacies are established to cater to the special or specified category of peoples like government officers, legislatures, patients from special clinics, etc. So, it distributes drugs to both inpatients and special outpatients. However, these pharmacies will have a lesser stock compared to the main pharmacy, which receives its supply in bulk from hospital stores.

The major advantage of satellite pharmacy service is that the patients are able to get the medicine quickly without spending much time. Moreover, the large crowd gathering in front of the main pharmacy and consequent problems are avoided.

The disadvantage is an increase in inventory and the subsequent cost. Nevertheless, almost all the problems in dispensing to inpatients are more or less solved in this method. Hence, modern or renovated old hospitals are equipped with satellite pharmacies, e.g. Rajiv Gandhi Government General Hospital, Chennai.

Charging of the Prescribed Drug

There are several methods for collecting money from the patients for the drug supplied to them. They are,

1. Direct payment by patients as done in private hospitals.

2. Payment by a third party like an insurance company.

3. Payment through subscription as in Employees State Insurance [ESI] scheme.

1. Direct payment

In this method, the cost of medicine is calculated either by the pharmacist or the accountant and collected by the hospital cashier. After the payment is made, the patient has to produce the receipt or bill to the pharmacist who then dispenses the medicines for which payment has been made. This method is followed in all the private hospitals and in some government hospitals as well for a specific category of patients.

2. Payment by the third party

In this method, a third party like an insurance company pays the charges for the medicines prescribed if the patient qualifies for the medical/health insurance policy. As per some company policies, the patient has to pay to the hospital first and gets reimbursement from the insurance company later after producing the bills, prescriptions and other documents required by the insurance company. But for some patients, instead of the insurance company, employers may be paying for their employee as per service agreements. In this method, the patients need not pay for their own medicines.

3. Payment through subscription

This is a method in which a fixed amount as the monthly or yearly subscription is deducted from the salaries of the employees by the employers and paid to the authorities specially arranged for giving treatment like Employees State Insurance (ESI) Corporation.

Under this scheme, the family members and the dependents of the employee are also eligible to receive treatment and medicines from ESI hospitals without paying. However, even if the employee or their dependents are not receiving any treatment in these hospitals, they still have to pay the subscription fee to the corporation every month. A part of the expenses for these hospitals is borne by the employers also, as welfare measures for their employees.

Pricing Policy

In all the above methods, the drugs are priced with a little margin of profit by the hospitals concerned. The percentage of margin differs in various hospitals. As a rule, the breakeven point is fixed as the price i.e., no loss, no profit price is charged from the patients.

Dispensing of Narcotics or Controlled Substances

During the course of dispensing to the patients, the pharmacist has to dispense narcotic drugs as well. Narcotics are the drugs that produce deleterious effects such as undue depression or stimulation of the human brain resulting in effects like euphoria, personality destabilizing effects, addiction, etc. Hence, there are certain conditions and procedures to dispense such drugs enforced by the government through the drugs control department. These procedures must be known to all dispensing pharmacists and they are expected to follow those guidelines in letter and spirit. Failing this may result in prosecution by the drugs inspectors and police personals.

Let us look at the general conditions for dispensing narcotics, followed by the specific procedures to be considered by the pharmacists while dispensing to outpatients and inpatients of a hospital.

General Conditions

1. No narcotic drug should be dispensed without a written prescription of a registered medical practitioner.

2. Narcotic drugs should not be dispensed for more than one day use unless specifically prescribed by the physician.

3. Narcotic prescriptions should be retained in the pharmacy after dispensing the drug or returned to the patient after putting the rubber stamp 'issued/dispensed' along with the signature (with date) of the pharmacist on the prescription. If retained, the prescriptions must be kept in a separate file for inspection by drug inspectors.

4. No prescription for narcotics may be refilled. If the procedure mentioned in point 3 is properly followed, no prescription with a refilling requirement will be seen in the pharmacy.

5. No controlled substance (narcotic) may be dispensed other than for a medical purpose.

6. Prescription for narcotics must be written in ink and shall not bear any erasing or alteration. It must be signed by the doctor along with their name and registration number rubber stamp.

7. Prescriptions for narcotics must be complete in all aspects, that is, they must contain full address and diagnosis of the patient as well as doctor's hospital address and phone number.

Hospital Procedure for Dispensing Narcotics

1. Responsibility for narcotics in the hospital

In general, the administrative head of the hospital is responsible for proper safeguarding and handling of the narcotics within the hospital. The chief pharmacist is responsible for the purchase, storage, and maintenance of accounts and proper dispensing of narcotics in particular. Similarly, the head nurse of the ward is responsible for the proper storage and use of controlled substances (narcotics) in the ward.

2. Dispensing to inpatients

The administration of narcotic drugs to the inpatients is carried out by the nurses and these drugs are not given directly to the patient for self-administration. There is always a greater control over its use as compared to the outpatients.

Hence, the procedure is simple. A separate copy of prescription should be written for narcotics for inpatients along with the usual prescription written on the case sheet by the treating physician. This separate prescription must be completed in all aspects as described above and sent to the dispensary. The drugs supplied are kept locked and the ward nurse has the access to it when it needs to be administered to the patient as per the directions written on the case sheet.

A pro re nata (prn) (occasionally) or si opus sit (SOS) (whenever necessary) prescriptions for narcotics must be discouraged except under special circumstances. The doctor may give orders by telephone in case of an emergency. Then, the nurse writes the order on the doctor's prescription sheet, clearly stating that it is a telephone order. The nurse has to write the doctor's name and also put her own initials. The doctor must then sign the order within 24 hours. Similarly, a doctor may give verbal order for narcotic drugs in an extreme emergency where time does not permit writing the order. The nurse must write the order on the prescription sheet and the doctor should sign it within 24 hours.

The doctor should not write a prescription for narcotics for their own use. Narcotics obtained for the ward use should not be issued to home use by the patients on discharge. These are all the procedures followed in the majority of the hospitals but may have additional or reduced conditions in a few hospitals.

3.   Dispensing to outpatients

The prescription for narcotics to outpatients must contain the following information:

(a)   Patient's full name

(b)   Patient address

(c)   Hospital number

(d)   Date

(e)   Name and strength of the drug

(f)   Quantity to be dispensed

(g)   Directions for use

(h)   Signature of the physician

The prescription must be written in ink and must not bear any correction. Narcotics should not be dispensed for more than one day use unless prescribed otherwise by the physician. Automatic stop order for narcotics after one day use is enforced by many hospitals in this regard. All the other general conditions for dispensing narcotics are applicable to the dispensing of narcotics to outpatients.

QUESTIONS

1. Who is an ambulatory patient?
2. Write a note on a mobile pharmacy.
3. Write briefly about satellite pharmacy.
4. Write short notes on the unit dose system.
5. Write an essay about dispensing to inpatients.
6. Explain the charging of prescribed drugs.
7. Detail the procedure to be followed for dispensing narcotics.
8. Describe the complete floor stock system and its advantages and disadvantages.

HOSPITAL FORMULARY

LEARNING OBJECTIVE

The Aim, Content, Preparation, Format, Appearance and Advantages and Disadvantages of a Hospital Formulary are explained in this chapter with an objective of conveying its importance to the students. The guiding principles to include or exclude a drug in the formulary is also given, thus the student will have a fairly large idea about Hospital Formulary on completion of this chapter.

INTRODUCTION

The hospital formulary is nothing but the hospital's own pharmacopeia. Now, the question is, why does a hospital need its own pharmacopeia when the government publishes pharmacopoeia for the entire country? Let's look at some of the strong arguments in favor:

1. A national Pharmacopoeia is big in volume. It contains monographs for a lot of drugs for which the government fix standards. However, a hospital does not necessarily need a long list of drugs.

2. It cannot be used as a ready reference in a hospital set up where information about a drug may be required on the spot and it cannot be made available to everybody.

3. The pharmacopoeia does not contain all the formulations used by the hospital which are separately published in books like National Formulary, Pharmaceutical codex, etc.

4. The pharmacopoeia does not contain all the information required by different health care professionals like nurses, dieticians, and laboratory technicians.

5. Since India was part of the British Empire in the last two centuries, the British pharmacopoeia was the official one in India and it had to be imported to India. It was not available throughout our country and that's when the need for preparing personalized pharmacopoeia arrived.

6. Due to the tremendous growth of science in the early 20th century, there came thousands of drug formulations into the market with claims of unproven efficacy and safety. The doctors were confused with these claims and counterclaims. The aggressive marketing technique adopted by pharmaceutical manufacturers was not helping either. There was a need for someone to verify the claim, find worth and safe formulation and recommend it to the physicians. The hospital management also found it very difficult to stock all the formulations prescribed by all its doctors.

Hence, hospital formulary comes into the picture. It contains the list of drugs approved by the hospital concerned. It was prepared by the expert members of the committee formed by the PTC of the hospital. The objective, content, and other details about the hospital formulary are discussed below.

Objectives

The ultimate aim of publishing a hospital formulary is to give the best treatment to the patient at a lower cost. The hospital formulary, as a book, has the following objectives.

It provides information on:

1. The name and other details about the drugs approved by the Hospital (to be prescribed to the patients of the particular hospital).

2. Hospital policies and procedures on the use of the above drugs and

3. General Information such as dosing rules, abbreviations, etc.

Content

The contents of the formulary are arranged under three main sections:

Section 1: Introduction (Policies and Procedures)

Section 2: List of Drugs

Section 3: Additional Information

Section 1: Introduction (Policies and Procedures)

In this section, the details about the Pharmacy and Therapeutics Committee, the name of its members, their designation, and official addresses are given. Furthermore, there are details of the sub-committee or the special committee that prepared the formulary, followed by the duties and responsibilities given to the various members of the sub-committee. It is further followed by the guidelines on instructions for using the formulary, interpretation, meaning, and legal limitations of its content. There are multiple references to sources of detailed information on formulary drugs, such as Pharmacopoeias, National Formularies and Hospital's own Drugs Information services.

As the formulary is binding in nature to the medical and paramedical staff of the hospital, it contains all the policies of the hospital with reference to the use of drugs. For example, it describes hospital regulations governing the prescribing, dispensing, and administering of drugs.

It also explains the rules regarding the prescription of controlled (Narcotic) drugs, automatic stop order, verbal drug orders, use of drug samples, reporting ADR and medication errors, etc.

The pharmacy operating procedures like working hours of various pharmacy wings of the hospital, outpatient services, inpatient services, pharmacy charging system, drug information services, etc, are also included in this premiere of the hospital formulary so as to ensure a tussle-free and smooth functioning of the hospital.

Section 2: List of Drugs

This section is the heart of the formulary. It lists the entire range of drugs and formulations approved by the hospital for prescribing to the patients of the hospital. They can be arranged under any one of the following methods.

1. Drugs under generic names arranged alphabetically.

2. Drugs under generic names arranged alphabetically but within the therapeutic classification.

3. A combination of the above two where the majority of the drugs are arranged according to the first method and a few therapeutic classes like ophthalmic drugs, otic drugs, dermatological preparations, etc are separately printed, while the drugs under the generic name are listed alphabetically in each of the above special sections.

As the elaborating the information about each drug is not possible and will defeat the very purpose of a book for ready reference, the formulary contains minimum essential information on each drug. They are:

1. Generic Name, if not available, as in the case of formulations, the common name or even the trade name.

2. Synonym, if any.

3. Dosage forms, strengths, packages and sizes, commonly stocked in the hospital's pharmacy.

4. The formula, if it is a combination product.

5. Dose (adult, children, and pediatric) and

6. Special instructions/precautions.

Section 3: Additional Information

The hospital formulary is prepared to guide and help the entire health care team of the hospital. Hence, it contains information useful for nurses, dieticians, lab technicians, and other public health workers. The following sums up the wealth of information available in a hospital formulary:

1. Posology (including methods of calculating doses)

2. Pediatric doses

3. Poisons and antidotes

4. Important laboratory values

5. Nutrition and calorific values

6. Height and weight chart

7. Immunization schedule
8. Diagnostic and pathological reagents
9. List of hospital approved abbreviations and
10. General and pharmacological index

Guiding Principles to Include or Exclude a Drug in the Formulary

One of the most difficult tasks of the pharmacy and therapeutic committee is the selection of drugs to include in the formulary. This is difficult because no member of the sub-committee formed for the purpose of preparation of formulary is experienced enough in all the fields of therapy. Hence, the committee always invites specialists from a particular field to its meetings to make a decision about the group of drugs used or available in a particular field. Thus, the experts, as well as the hospital staff's own experience, is the very first, undisputable guideline to include or exclude a particular drug in the formulary.

The second criterion is the inclusion of a particular drug or formulation in other books of a standard like Pharmacopoeias, National formularies, etc.

The third one is the manufacturer of a particular drug must have proven integrity, dependability, and track record.

The fourth one is the product in question must be approved, accepted, and in the market for a long time.

The fifth one is the drug or formulation must declare all its content in the label and no secret composition is acceptable to the committee.

The sixth principle is that the drug or formulation must comply with all the legal requirements of Drugs and Cosmetic Act and Rules.

If the drug, after approval and inclusion in the formulary is found to be deficient in any one of the above principles, it will be deleted from the formulary by suitable notification or circular by the PTC.

The above principles may be published in the hospital formulary itself and circulated among the staff of the hospital. This way the staff acquires an understanding as to why a particular drug is not found or left out from the formulary. Also, it encourages the staff concerned to recommend a particular drug to the PTC if it meets all the above guiding principles.

Preparation of the Formulary

When the PTC of the hospital decides to prepare and adopt a formulary for the hospital concerned, they constitute a subcommittee for the purpose. The director or the chief of the pharmacy services of the hospital is given the responsibility for preparing the formulary with the active participation and co-operation of all the members of the sub-committee.

The sub-committee is briefed on the series of rules or guidelines (refer above) to evaluate drugs for admission to the formulary and also on the content and format by PTC. If the PTC decides to have only a drug list or catalog for use in the hospital instead of a full formulary, the same is conveyed to the subcommittee which prepares the one on demand. However, there are many differences between a formulary and a mere drug list.

A formulary is more informative in nature. Its contents range from the generic name of the drugs to posology, poisons, antidotes, and the data required by nurses, dieticians, and lab technicians. On the other hand, a drug list or catalog contains only the name of the drug and dose range.

Thus, the formulary has an informative, educative role and hence is useful to trainee doctors, nurses, and pharmacists. However, the preparation, maintenance, and updating of the drug list or catalog are easier as compared to the formulary. Additions and deletions are easily made to the list, whereas, it requires a lot of effort, time, and cost to update a formulary.

Any additional information about a drug in the list can be obtained only by referring to suitable sources like books, manufacturer's literature or internet or drug information centers. But the formulary gives adequate, essential information about each drug in a nutshell.

Format and Appearance

As the formulary is for ready reference on a daily basis, its format is very important. Looking at the previously published formularies of other hospitals within the country or abroad, it gives an idea to develop the one suitable for local conditions. The formulary published by the Vellore Christian Medical College (CMC) hospital in Tamil Nadu offers a remarkable model for the others. The National Formulary of India (NFI) published by Government of India is equally useful as a forerunner.

Size: Experience has shown that a formulary which is sufficiently small in size to fit into the apron or clinical/lab coat will enjoy the acceptance of all concerned. Thus, the size of 10 cm × 18 cm is widely accepted.

Appearance: Each section of the formulary can be printed in different color papers, thus helping the users to locate the particular section quicker. The poisons and antidotes section, for example, can be printed on pink-colored paper while a pediatric section can exhibit a light green color. The laboratory values can exhibit a blue color, and so on. Alternatively, 'edge index' can also be used for the same purpose but that will make the production cost go up marginally.

Since the formulary is to be used often and carried daily, good bound volumes should be prepared with covers ranging from paper and cardboard to plastic or leather binding. At the same time, the formulary should be printed on good quality paper in order to reduce its overall weight to carry in coat pockets easily.

Moreover, the hospital formulary must be updated and revised as often as possible or necessary. Usually, the formulary is updated once in a year. In the meantime, supplements may be published in between the editions.

Distribution of Formulary

Formulary should be distributed to the following people and places of the hospital.

  1. All the Doctors employed in the hospital

2. All the wards of the hospital

3. All the Heads of the Department who are related to patient care.

4. Outpatient Department (OPD) and emergency room (causality)

5. All the sections of hospital pharmacy including stores and Drug Information Center and

6. The administrative office of the hospital.

The hospital formulary copies can be sent to the higher authorities like Pharmacy Council of India, State Pharmacy Council, Director of Medical Education, Director of Medical and Public Health Services, Director of Drugs Control and to the Library of University of Health Sciences.

Advantages and Disadvantages of Hospital Formulary

Advantages

1. Patients are assured of safe and rational drug therapy.

2. The treatment given to them costs less, compared to the treatment with irrational and expensive drugs or drugs with doubtful benefits.

Disadvantages

1. It restricts the doctors' freedom to prescribe drugs of their choice.

2. If the formulary is not updated regularly, new and effective drugs arrived cannot be prescribed to patients.

3. If the guiding principle for including or excluding a drug in the hospital formulary is not followed strictly, there are chances of unwanted drugs entering into the formulary and the deserving drugs getting left out of the formulary. This results in the defeating of the very purpose of hospital formulary.

Nevertheless, the hospital formulary system is the most useful one in a populated country like India.

QUESTIONS

1. What is a hospital formulary?

2. What are the objectives of a hospital formulary?

3. Discuss the advantages and disadvantages of a hospital formulary.

4. Explain the content of a hospital formulary.

5. What are the criteria for selecting a drug to include in the hospital formulary?

6. What are the guiding principles to prepare a Hospital formulary?

7. How do hospital formularies differ from Pharmacopeia? Explain the format and appearance of the Hospital Formulary.

CHAPTER 7

THERAPEUTIC DRUG MONITORING

LEARNING OBJECTIVE

The chapter aims to provide fairly good knowledge about an important function of a Clinical pharmacist. It explains the need for TDM, Factors to be considered during TDM, Development of TDM Services and Problems in TDM. On learning these, the student will be in a position to accept these works during his practice. To further improve his understanding of the task the Indian scenario of TDM is also given at the end of the chapter.

Therapeutic Drug Monitoring [TDM] is a process of monitoring drugs given to patients by measuring the drug concentration in the patient's body fluids and analyzing other vital parameters.

NEED FOR TDM

It is one of the most important aspects of drug therapy review to monitor the drugs used in therapy. It is done by analyzing the body fluids of the patient regularly on a periodic basis. Based on the pharmacokinetics of the drug used on the particular patient, critical clinical decisions are made. The drug concentration in the body fluids of an individual patient is used to determine an optimum drug regimen for that patient. The ideal therapy can be given to a patient only by individualization of dose and drug regimen and the only way to go about it is proper TDM.

Factors to be considered during TDM

TDM is not meant all drugs and cannot be undertaken for all the patients. Not to mention, this task is next to impossible and unnecessary. The cost incurred during the process is one of the major prohibitory factors. Hence, we have to be selective regarding the drugs that require TDM. The criteria for selecting such drugs are outlined below:

1. **Drugs with narrow therapeutic index:** Therapeutic index can be defined as the difference between a safe therapeutic dose and a toxic one. Wider the difference, safer will be the drug. However, if there is a narrow difference between the two doses, the drug has to be used with caution. In order to arrive at a correct dose that produces the desired effect and also to prevent it from reaching toxic concentration, therapeutic drug monitoring should be done. For example, drugs like, aminoglycosides, antineoplastic drugs, and cardiac glycosides must be monitored by TDM.

2. **Drugs with varying pharmacokinetic properties:** The amount of drug which reaches the systemic circulation- the bioavailability, differs not only among the drugs but also varies in individuals, and different dosage forms of the same drug. Hence, the need for monitoring such drugs. Absorption, distribution, metabolism, and excretion of these drugs play a major role in the variation of bioavailability of them in individual patients.

3. **Drugs that produce different amounts of effect:** Some drugs produce a huge effect on some patients or very little effect on other patients for the same dose. This variation is due to many factors, one of them being the concentration of drug that reaches the site of action and the consequent effect it produces. There may or may not be a correlation between the amounts of drug at the site of action and inside the plasma. The other factors might include their protein binding on tissue protein and the diffusion rate through the membrane. This inter-individual variability in pharmacodynamic or the effect of drugs is one of the major complications of TDM. However, TDM also helps in identifying such cases. Therefore, the necessary precautions can be followed while treating such cases. A good example of this is Sodium valproate.

4. TDM is essential if the patient is not responding to a standard drug regimen for a considerable time.

5. This non-responsiveness to standard drugs may be due to non-compliance or drug resistance. In order to find out the real reason, TDM must be performed.

6. Many times, drug toxicity symptoms are mistaken for disease manifestations. For example, an increase in creatinine levels in the patients may be due to disease or graft rejection. Cyclosporine, which is used to suppress the patients' immunity, may produce this toxic effect and hence, TDM becomes a necessity for such drugs.

7. Some drugs produce huge effects even for a small increase in the dose. Such drugs are said to have non-linear kinetics in their actions. For example, Phenytoin produces a disproportionate effect for a small dose increase. These drugs should be monitored by TDM.

8. We know for sure that some drugs after reaching a toxic range in the body produce a series of side effects. Needless to mention, such drugs should be closely monitored.

9. If a drug's pharmacological effect cannot be measured by any means, it should be monitored without a second thought.

10.   Furthermore, drugs that are given to infants along with their reaction cases under extraordinary circumstances should be monitored.

11.   Pharmacokinetics of drugs is certainly altered in some cases. This is usually occurring in case of anemia, pregnancy, liver damage, kidney damage, etc. Hence, TDM is a must for these cases and conditions.

12.   Because of the non-availability of alternatives, we may have to administer the drugs which have the potential to interact. For example anti-T.B and antiepileptic drugs, if given together may interact and produce side effects. Even if a proper dosage interval between the drugs is taken into consideration, TDM must be undertaken to ensure the safety of the patient.

Thus, TDM has to be ordered by treating physicians for drugs like, digoxin, lithium, quinidine, propranolol, salicylates, phenobarbitone, theophylline, phenytoin, aminoglycosides, procainamide, and methotrexate.

Development of TDM Services

A. Organization: As the TDM involves services like sample collection, sample analysis, interpretation of results, and taking appropriate clinical and therapeutic decisions, specialists in all these fields must be employed. Thus, the services of a suitably trained physician, clinical pharmacologist, clinical biochemist, and clinical pharmacist are required to run an effective TDM service. Additionally, suitable analytical methods for sample analysis, expertise in analyzing those samples, producing results within a short period possible are also equally essential to perform TDM.

B. Functioning: First of all a treating physician must request for TDM services for the patient if the expected clinical results are not produced for standard or special drug regimen. Thereafter, the sample is drawn (usually body fluids) from the patient and analyzed by a clinical pharmacist or an analyst. With their knowledge in the pharmacokinetics of drugs, a clinical pharmacist is most suitable for this job and also to further interpret the results. Later on, the results are conveyed to the physician who requested the service, in writing, along with a clinical suggestion on the refinement of the current drug therapy. Note that the patient has to pay for the TDM service.

C. Information required for TDM service

1.   **Information about the patient:** All relevant information about the patient should be provided to the clinical pharmacist in order to interpret the results, calculate the dose, and suggest refinement to the therapy. Hence, not only the usual information like the patient's age, sex, height, and weight, but also other conditions like pharmacological status should be provided in the request to TDM service. If not provided, this information should be collected at the time of drawing a sample from the patient.

2.   **Sample time:** Usually, the sample is drawn at an appropriate time, depending on the body fluid to be collected like blood, urine, etc. If the blood is collected from the patient, it should be between two doses when the concentration is low. Also, the patient must be in a steady-state while drawing the sample. However, peak concentrations are to be measured in certain

cases like IV administration of antibiotics, theophylline, and antiarrhythmic drugs. This time of collection of the sample should be mentioned in the analytical records.

3. **Interpretation of blood drug concentration:** It is important to compare the plasma concentration with the therapeutic range for the given drug. If it is in excess, a reassessment should be carried out. In case, it is below the range, appropriate corrections should be made in the dose to bring levels closer to the equated range. For doing this, one should have knowledge and expertise in pharmacokinetics and pharmacodynamic. Moreover, the interpretation of results should be in light of the clinical situation of the patient, arrived at from the information provided.

Problems in TDM

1. **Analytical methods:** In order to save the cost, multiple assays of TDM are carried out using low-cost equipment or cheap methods. For instance, most of the assays are done using a Calorimeter or a Spectrophotometer rather than using an HPLC which is far more accurate. The drugs which produce fluorescent metabolites should not be analyzed using spectrofluorimetric methods, For example analysis of quinidine by spectrofluorimetric method gives twice the quantity of the result given by HPLC method.

   Similarly, Radio Immuno Assay (RIA) is a problem in measuring digoxin concentration. Some of the circulating natural substances in newborn infants show a positive result for quinidine concentration by RIA method, even though they are not given quinidine. Hence, the non-specific methods of analysis pose a major problem for TDM.

2. **Altered protein binding:** The protein binding of drugs and consequent free drug concentration in the blood depends on several factors. It is altered due to disease conditions. Hence, measuring plasma drug concentration becomes useless if not correlated with other measurements.

3. **Quality control problems:**

A. **Interferences with drug assay by other substances:** Combination of drugs is one of the major problems in analysis. For example, gentamicin with gallium, phenytoin with phenobarbitone and digoxin with prednisolone interfere in the analysis.

B. **Stereoisomer:** Several drugs are administered as a mixture of isomers. Although they are chemically the same compounds, they differ vastly in their pharmacological actions. Hence, a mere assay of a mixture of isomers will not help in determining the pharmacokinetics and pharmacodynamics of the drug. One example of this is Verapamil.

C. **Active metabolites:** Some of the metabolites are active, sometimes more than the parent drug, hence, TDM should assay both these compounds while deciding corrections in the regimen. One example of this case is Procainamide and its active metabolite. N-acetylprocainamide and 3-hydroxy quinidine and quinidine.

D. Many TDM assay results are not accurate or reproducible, making them difficult to rely upon.

4. Apart from this, factors that make the measurement of plasma concentration useless also affects the TDM. They are:

A. Drugs whose response is easily measurable, e.g. Diuretics, hypoglycemics

B. Drugs that are activated in the body, e.g. Levodopa.

C. 'Hit and Run' drugs, whose effects last much longer than the drug itself (e.g. Reserpine, MAO inhibitors) and

D. Drugs with irreversible action (e.g. Organophosphates and anti-cholinestarases)

INDIAN SCENARIO FOR T.D.M

The Therapeutic Drug Monitoring concept and practice have not been able to develop a firm root in India. There are many reasons for the same. To list a few, prohibitive cost, non-availability of facilities and convictions of treating physicians are on the forefront.

Cost Factor

In India, we have both the government sector and the private sector health facilities looking after the health care needs of the people. The former has limited resources to meet the extra expenses involved in TDM. With the limited budget allocation, the government hospitals are struggling to meet even the basic treatment expenses of thousands of people reaching out to them. The crowd coming to the government hospitals is increasing day by day without any corresponding increase in the monitory support by authorities. Hence, patients in government hospitals are rarely monitored therapeutically. Moreover Clinical pharmacists need to be appointed in those hospitals to perform those duties, that is yet to be done. If at all any TDM is performed on a patient in govt. hospital, it may be due to unavoidable need or interest by treating physicians.

On the other hand, TDM can be performed for the patients admitted to private hospitals where clinical pharmacists and facilities are available. The patients of private corporate hospitals can afford to bear the expenses to a certain extent. However, if the cost is exorbitantly high, the patients may tend to avoid these in the future. Hence, there are limitations to the use of TDM in both government and private hospitals. The only way to overcome such obstacles is by increasing the health care budget by our governments and also by implementing universal coverage of people with health insurance schemes.

Availabilities of Facilities

As mentioned above, government hospitals are not able to offer facilities for TDM services due to meager resources. However, these facilities are comparatively easier to establish as well as to maintain. The conventional analytical methods and equipment may not be much useful to perform TDM tests. The instruments and equipment required to serve the purpose must be modern (often imported). The cost of chemicals and reagents used in these procedures is also on the higher side. Hence, only limited facilities are established for the same. Although there are scores of suppliers of kits for TDM in India, most of them supply imported kits, the cost of which is naturally prohibitive to the process.

Apart from the above, not all the drugs administered to a patient can be monitored for want of reliable method of analysis. As we know the analysis of body fluids is much more difficult, complex and misleading than the other analytical samples. The samples are difficult to analyze because of interfering metabolites in the body fluids. Additionally, a great deal of this difficulty is also owed to the patients' lifestyle, habits and concurrent intake of allopathic medicines or medicines from alternative systems of medicine like Ayurveda, Siddha, Unani, and Homeopathy. Hence, the sample has to be collected from the patients admitted in the wards. Furthermore, the time of collection, the method, and the site of sample collection also influence the results. We need to have infallible facilities for all these tasks.

Conviction of Treating Physicians

To introduce and maintain TDM services in India, treating physicians need to be convinced for its importance and usability. The majority of Indian doctors believe that TDM is not an essential part of their treatment and it unnecessarily increases the cost and duration of the treatment. That apart, they have the hidden apprehension that if TDM detects anything unusual they may be held responsible. Hence, most of the physicians try to avoid TDM as far as possible. As long as it is not performed any untoward problem or unusual development in patients can be attributed to disease factors and not on the treatment. Hence, it requires a lot of conviction and faith by treating physicians that their services are to save and cure the patient in time without causing any trouble to anyone. The physicians must understand that going forward with a procedure like TDM will only help them grow as a health expert.

QUESTIONS

1. Define TDM

2. List the factors affecting TDM

3. How will you develop TDM services?

4. Write an essay about the selection of drugs for TDM

5. Describe the Indian scenario for T.D.M

MEDICATION ADHERENCE

LEARNING OBJECTIVE

By explaining the Definition, Evidence, Reasons, Results, and Remedy for Non-adherence the chapter convey a reasonable and working knowledge about the subject matter Non-Adherence. Hence while practicing the profession one may find it useful and that is the objective of the chapter.

INTRODUCTION

If the patients follow the instructions given by their doctors and pharmacists while under treatment, it is known as medication adherence or patient adherence. It mainly depends on the understanding of the patient and to a certain extent, the severity of the disease. When the disease or the troubling symptoms start receding after a few days of treatment, the patient's adherence also starts receding. The poor understanding of the instructions also leads to non-adherence.

DEFINITION

"Non-adherence is the situation where the patient is not following the instructions by health care team regarding diet, exercise, rest, return appointment, refilling in addition to the use of drugs, etc.".

The self-regulated dose of drugs, as in asthma, diabetes, etc, depending on the severity of the condition of the patient cannot be termed as non-adherence. It is also true in the case of intermittent treatment with analgesics. Non-adherence by the patients may be due to inadequate instructions by the doctor and pharmacist. They may fail to present the instructions in an understandable manner leading to confusion, in turn, non-adherence.

Evidence of Non-adherence or Monitoring of Patient Medication Adherence

Although the patients usually deny non-adherence, the following pieces of evidence point towards the situation of non-adherence which is easily detected by the pharmacists via simple monitoring of the patients.

The omission of a dose, error in dose, error in the time of administration and taking the drug for the wrong purpose, all comes under non-adherence. Also, the non-refilling the prescription in time and premature discontinuation of treatment are considered as pieces of evidence for non-adherence.

This situation is more among the outpatients because of the lack of supervision. It is also prevalent among pediatric and geriatric patients who cannot take their medicines on their own and depend on others for drug administration. This evidence can be used to device the methods of assessing non-adherence as well as the extent or level of non-adherence.

Methods of Assessing Non-adherence

The following are the various methods of assessing non-adherence:

1. Interrogation
2. Verification of left-out medicines on hand
3. Analysis of drugs in body fluids and
4. Use of markers

1. **Interrogation:** Patients can be thoroughly enquired about their adherence to various instructions by asking clever questions. It is one of the easiest methods. It does not involve any cost but its accuracy is doubtful because the patient may lie and hide the facts which cannot be verified. At the same time, it is not feasible to interrogate all the patients every time we suspect non-adherence. Hence, other methods must be taken into consideration.

2. **Verification of balance drugs with the patient:** It is possible to verify the residual medicines available with the patient (excess or less) so as to detect non-adherence. However, it requires efforts as well as money as the patient has to go home and bring the remaining drugs. Therefore, the accuracy of the method is doubtful.

3. **Analysis of drugs in body fluids:** It is a feasible and accurate method, however, it is costlier compared to the previous two methods. To analyze the sample, the services of analyst, chemicals, procedures, and equipment are needed. By this method, only the previous dose can be verified and not the doses of previous days.

4. **Use of markers:** Some marker compounds are added to the drugs so that they can be identified in the urine of the patient. The absence of such markers indicates non-adherence by the patient. Although it is a very accurate method, it has almost nil feasibility and the cost involved is also prohibitive.

Though so many methods are available to assess non-adherence, they are not much used because it is understood that complying with the instructions is the responsibility of the patient. If any drug is to be administered on priority and non-adherence may lead to severe consequences to the patient as well as to the society, then the patients are admitted in the ward or quarantined, This usually happens in the case of infectious diseases. The drugs are administered by nurses or doctors regularly.

In order to assess the seriousness of the problem, the level of adherence to the instructions must be calculated. It is calculated using the following formula:

$$\text{Percentage adherence} = \frac{\text{NDP} - \text{NME}}{\text{NDP}} \times 100$$

Where NDP is the number of doses prescribed,

NME is the number of medication errors.

Note that less than 90% adherence is not acceptable. So, it is important to figure out the reasons for non- adherence before finding out the results and remedy for the problem.

Causes of Non-adherence

There are many factors responsible for non-adherence. They can be classified into the following categories:

1. Disease factors

2. Treatment factors

3. Medicine factors and

4. Health professional factors

1. **Diseases factors:** Non-adherence depends on the diseases which require long time treatment like TB. After faithfully following the instructions for some time, patients start drifting willingly or unwillingly. However, if the consequences of discontinuing the therapy are brought to their knowledge, they are motivated to adhere to the instructions. Some diseases subside after a few days of treatment and the symptoms disappear and hence, the patients assume that they are cured and stop taking drugs. The problem is further worsened by a lack of symptoms even after discontinuation of the drugs. Thus, disease factor plays a major role in non- adherence.

2. **Treatment factors:** Some doctors prescribe multiple drugs for the treatment which leads to non-adherence. The patients either forget one or the other drug or willingly stop any of them as per their convenience. Hence, non-essential drugs should not be prescribed. Again, if similar-looking drugs are prescribed to the patients, they get confused and stop taking them or take a double dose of the same drug by mistake. A careful prescription can prevent this problem.

Another major problem with the treatment is the frequency of the dose with single or multiple drugs. There are high chances of missing any of the doses in the course of a day. Higher the frequency of a dose, the higher are the chances of non-adherence. Hence, the prescriber must go for once a day (sustained-release) formulations and combination drugs. Moreover, the treatment must be finished as quickly as possible. This doesn't mean a doctor should prescribe a highly potent drug for simple ailment.

3. **Medicine factors:** The medicines prescribed to the patient should be acceptable to them. Any inconvenience in the intake of any of the drug prescribed should be brought to the notice of the doctor or the pharmacist. Following this, the particular drug should be substituted with a more suitable but equally potent drug. For example, the nature of medicine prescribed may disappoint the patient leading to non-adherence. The unpleasant taste of liquid medicines, inappropriate package, poor labeling, staining ointments, very big size of the tablet, painful injections all leads to non-adherence.

Moreover, the cost of medicine is also an important contributory factor for non-adherence. If the drugs that are often prescribed are very expensive, the patient might try to change the doctor rather than adhering to their prescription.

The adverse drug effects of a prescribed medicine are another discouraging factor. If the patient feels sleepy throughout the day or if they know drugs like antipsychotics lead to impotence, they will stop taking them. Any amount of counseling will be insignificant help in those matters.

4. **Health professionals factors:** Sometimes, the instructions given to the patient may not be understandable and there is a chance that they may fail to comprehend the importance of the therapy. In such cases, they definitely slip to non-adherence. For example, there should not be any uncertainty in the instructions given to the patient. 'If' and 'buts', 'as directed', 'whenever necessary' are all such instructions that make the patients indecisive of the drug intake.

If the patients are made to wait for a long time to see the doctor or the pharmacist, they sometimes leave without waiting any further and take the drugs as they like or understand. They are not likely to come back even at a later date fearing the long waiting period. This is the reason why many doctors are disposing of the cases with quick diagnosis and prescription. Most of the occasions, they don't have the time to counsel the patients or to explain the importance of each drug. Thus, the health professionals are also responsible for non-adherence by the patient.

Results of Non-adherence

There are many consequences of non-adherence and many are interrelated as well. For instance, non-adherence first results in underutilization of drugs which not only deprives the patient of any therapeutic benefit but also leads to the recurrence of infection. Once relapsed, the infection may not respond to the earlier drug due to the development of resistance by the microorganism. There are multiple examples of resistant microorganisms like Tubercle bacilli and malarial parasite that do not respond to Isoniazid and Chloroquine respectively. These resistance organisms are dangerous to the patient as well as the people in closer proximity.

The situation warrants large doses of present medicament or more potent medicament than the current one. Therefore, patients are exposed to greater risks. The problem does not end here. Underutilization of one drug may result in an excessive response to other drugs used simultaneously. For example, if Digoxin, Furosemide, and Potassium chloride tablets are prescribed and the patient fails to take the Potassium Chloride tablet, it leads to the more toxic effect of Digoxin.

Similarly, the overutilization of drugs is also dangerous due to the risk of side effects. Some patients forget one dose and double the next dose to make up for the loss. Some others think if one tablet gives so much relief, taking multiple tablets at the same time would only increase the benefits. Such patients should be educated to make them aware of the flaws in this logic.

The unused drugs lying in the patient's home leads to the following problems:

(a)   They may be used inappropriately at a later date.

(b)   Their storage condition is questionable.

(c)   They may be used accidentally later and

(d)   They may be consumed to commit suicide or used for harming someone else.

Thus, non-adherence is not a simple problem as many would think. It is a serious problem and hence, the doctors, nurses, and pharmacists must pay the required attention.

Remedy for Non-adherence- Pharmacist's Role

Now that we have an idea of how serious the problem is, let us discuss the ways and means of tackling it. Non-adherence as such cannot be totally eradicated. At best, adherence can be improved. If the reasons or factors for non-adherence are identified and removed, it leads to better adherence.

All the patients are viewed as potential non-compliers and we must identify the cause of non-adherence in order to find a solution. The simplification of regimen is one of the best solutions for the problem. If fewer drugs and fewer doses are prescribed, half of the problem will be over.

Patient education is another important tool to achieve better adherence. This can be given to the patient via counseling.

During counseling:

(a)   The patient should be made aware that they have been diagnosed with a sickness.

(b)   They should be educated on the consequences of that disease.

(c)   They should be thoroughly informed how the treatment will reduce the present or future severity of the disease

(d)   They should be explained how the cost of treatment and other disadvantages are insignificant, considering the benefits of the regimen.

If counseling on the above lines is carried out for the non-compliers or potential non-compliers, it results in better and successful treatment.

Moreover, high standards of dispensing also help in better adherence by the patient, as many of their doubts are cleared by the process. For example, if supplementary labels, warning cards, booklets, leaflets, and calendar packing are used while dispensing, patients appreciate it and fall in line with the instructions by the pharmacist. But, at the same time, excessive information given to a patient may lead to self-medication or even treatment of dependants at a later period. This must be kept in mind while counseling for adherence.

CONCLUSION

As pointed out in the foregoing pages, non-adherence is prevalent among outpatients only. By the very nature of their disease, the treatment may be for a short period or even if it is for a longer period, their diseases may be of such nature they need not be admitted to the hospital. Only the latter cases have to be monitored by the pharmacist for non-adherence. Examples for these cases are diabetics, hypertension, epilepsy, cardiac diseases, TB, asthma, leprosy, etc. The condition worsens due to various reasons, one being is non-adherence. The pharmacists are advised to look for such non-compliers and to take suitable action as detailed above.

QUESTIONS

1. Define non-adherence.

2. List the methods of assessing non-adherence.

3. Write a note on the effect of non-adherence.

4. How can you tackle the problem of non-adherence?

5. Write an essay about non-adherence, its effects, and reasons.

6. What are the factors affecting adherence? How it is solved?

7. Explain the methods of detecting non-adherence. How will you calculate the extent or level of non-adherence?

8. Describe the role of a pharmacist in medication adherence.

9. How will you monitor patients for medication adherence?

CHAPTER 9

PATIENT MEDICATION HISTORY INTERVIEW

LEARNING OBJECTIVE

Almost complete detail is given about an appreciable job of a pharmacist—Conducting medication history interview--in this chapter. Hence on concluding the reading and understanding of the chapter the reader will acquire the skill and competence to conduct this interview. The finer aspects of an interview are explained with sample questions. The benefit of medication history interview is explained at the end of the chapter

INTRODUCTION

At the outset, the clinical pharmacist must keep it in mind that this is not an interview of a candidate for a job or place in an institution. They must remember that they are going to interview a patient who is sick, anxious, and not in a position to oblige, regardless of the intention. Hence, the interview must be planned in such a way as to get maximum information with minimum trouble and time to the patient. Moreover, the clinical pharmacist must remember that their approach must be in a manner that the patient should not feel that they are being questioned by someone superior. At no point, the patient should feel that they are under pressure to disclose personal information and other details.

Difference between Interview and Counseling

A clinical pharmacist has to interact with the patient from the very beginning of a patient's stay in the hospital to their discharge from the ward. They have to interact with the patient on multiple occasions, from the date of admission in the ward to the end of treatment and even beyond that. During these interactions, the initial days are reserved for gathering information about the patient. The later stages involve informing the patients about their post-hospital routines. Generally, the "information gathering" is known as an interview and "information giving" is termed as counseling. However, there is no hard and fast rule that there should be a fixed pattern to conduct this procedure. These processes may interchange in some situations where the information is given during the interview and gathered in the counseling sessions.

Need for Patient Medication History Interview

If an interview is conducted properly and all the relevant information is obtained from the patient, the medical fraternity is enormously benefitted. The advantages are numerous and beneficial to all the people involved in the healthcare of the patient, including the patient themselves. It helps in speedy and correct diagnosis. It avoids unnecessary repetitions of earlier ineffective treatment; it saves the patient from unpleasant exposure to drugs allergic to them; it also prevents a patient from ADR, drug interaction, etc.

Furthermore, it gives an idea about the patient's habits, weaknesses, dependencies, and other requirements. Hence, clinical pharmacists can effectively monitor drug therapy later or modify drug therapy to suit the requirements of the patient. Without prior medication history of the patient on hand, these things are not possible and it may be too late to have this kind of data at a later stage.

To summarize the need or advantages, the patient interview opens the possibility for the best treatment and consequent reduction in time, energy, and money involved in the treatment.

Pre-requirements for an Interview

The patient who is to be interviewed by the pharmacist might have had the same or some other disease earlier and that illness experience and the present mood bring in a lot of stress on the patient. Hence, you cannot expect an outright co-operation from the patient. If someone gets sick in our family, not only the patient but the entire family is worried. All routine errands of all family members get disturbed in case the patient is the breadwinner of the family. These patients are more worried about expenses and loss of income than the disease itself. Moreover, they tend to exaggerate everything in their minds.

They are highly likely to develop worries about permanent disability, helplessness, and even death. Hence, a Clinical pharmacist must be sympathetic and helpful to the patient so that they can cope with the situation. This is the most important pre-requisite for a medication history interview.

The success of an interview depends on the pharmacist's approach. They must start the interview with as much information about the patient as in their possession. They are expected to know the patient's name, age, and present complaint from the hospital records. Also, they should know the physical condition of the patient like whether the patient is in acute pain, conscious, and communicative. Usually, the patients are admitted to the wards after first aid, essential clinical procedures in the outpatient department (OPD), or other emergencies. The pharmacist must verify all the possible situations and then they can safely assume that the patient may be in a position to answer the questions during the interview. Similarly, knowing the probable diagnosis may help in providing some idea about the severity of the disease, the possible diagnostic procedures ahead, etc. Thus, a thorough preparation before the interview is a pre-requisite for an interview.

Forms of Medication Interview or Structure of Patient's Case History

The patient's medication history and its content are discussed below in detail. Let us first summarize the structure.

- Patient's name, age, sex, and address
- Date of admission and the patient's hospital registration number
- Present complaint
- Already existing diseases like, T.B, Asthma, Diabetes, etc.
- Medicines currently in taking [Prescription and OTC drugs with dose used]
- Use of drugs of alternative systems medicine like Siddha, Ayurveda, etc.
- Allergy to the drug, food, and other things
- Problems encountered, if any, during drug use [ADR, Drug Interaction]
- Immunization [if relevant]
- Pregnancy and related problems [if applicable]
- Any previous surgery and its current status
- Social drug use habits [alcohol, tobacco etc.]
- Any evidence of drug abuse or misuse
- The general attitude towards the use of medicine [compliance/ noncompliance]
- Patient's opinion for present illness.

As mentioned earlier, all the above information cannot be obtained in one sitting by the Clinical Pharmacist. It is important to follow up to get the remaining information. For example, the patient may not remember the name of the medicine they already used for their present or past illness. A piece of information like this has to be gathered from their old prescriptions, discharge notes, bills of community pharmacies or by looking at the unused balance medicines. They can also directly contact the community pharmacist where the patient used to purchase medicines. By all means, the clinical pharmacist must try to get the full information listed above by clever questioning and efforts during medication history interview. Only a complete and comprehensive interview will serve its purpose of ensuring correct, quick and cost-effective therapy for the patient and help the hospital authorities to conduct an effective Drug Utilization Evaluation [DUE] later.

How to conduct a useful Interview?

The interview should be started with a polite introduction which leads to a long term relationship and rapport between the pharmacist and the patient. The medication history interview is not an exemption to this. The clinical pharmacist must open the interview with self-introduction after verification of the patient's identity. This must be followed by defining their role as an interviewer, the purpose, approximate time required for the interview, and other basic details. This helps in bringing the patient's mood to normal and they are inclined to co-operate. Then without going for specific details, their general daily routines, hobbies and social history like neighborhood environment, etc. can be enquired.

Once this preliminary part of the interview is over, the pharmacist should use their communication skills to get complete and correct information about the medication history. They should get the details about the prescribed and non-prescribed medicines currently taken by the patient. They should also gather information regarding the previous diseases or any current chronic diseases under treatment, allergies or problems with adverse effects, and possible drug misuse. All this information will not come up right away. The pharmacist must present the questions smartly, some open questions maybe and some would be closed questions.

Open questions are those for which patients can give lengthy, descriptive answers and the closed questions are required to be answered with a simple 'yes' or 'no'. The closed questions don't offer any opportunity to the patient to avoid or circumvent the answer and hence, should be used judiciously without offending the patient. If offended, proceeding further with the interview will be a waste of time. It might be a complete failure as the patient's co-operation ends with their hurt personality.

However, careful questioning will not lead to such an unpleasant end. Hence, the pharmacist must be attuned to the types of questions asked, the manner in which the questions are asked, and avoid repetitions. The technical terms should be avoided as much as possible or explained if absolutely necessary.

Usually, the patients have a mental setup that if a person is willing to listen, they should open up about all their problems and feelings. The pharmacist must make use of this mentality of the patients to gather the information needed. They should smartly handle the patient and make sure they share the real body problems without much interruption.

This apart, a successful interview requires the use of correct body language by the interviewer. The right body language increases the success chances of the interview.

Role of Body Language

In order to communicate effectively with others, body language plays an important role. Just like words, your body also sends messages to people. Communicating with deaf and dumb people via sign language is an example of this. When a message is delivered with facial expressions, hand gestures, and other body movements and postures, it reaches to the receiver quickly. Often, the pharmacists use it rather than sitting idly, giving blanks looks to the patients.

Making eye contact with the patients while they speak, head nods and inclining towards them are some of the signs of the body which indicate that the pharmacist is actively listening to the patient. Similarly, even the voice of the pharmacist while speaking to the patient has a significant role. The tone and tempo of the voice convey the message that one is sympathetic towards others. A voice filled with concern will definitely influence the patient. Thus, a sweet empathetic voice is of great help to the pharmacist to achieve what they want out of the interview.

Role of Prompts

Irrespective of the pharmacist's sympathetic behavior and good body language, all the needed information from the patient cannot be obtained due to multiple reasons. Few among them are patient's forgetfulness, lack of concentration or ignorance about the medicine they are taking and its usage. It is more acute in the case of illiterate and semi-literate patients. They may not be able to answer the pharmacist's questions accurately as such that the medication history interview may not be useful.

In such situations, the interviewing pharmacist has to adopt a few techniques like prompting or getting help from the family members of the patient. Prompting is nothing but stimulating or leading a person to start and sustain something. The pharmacist can ask prompting questions so that the patient starts recollecting the answer to the questions. Prompting helps trigger the patient's memory. For example, the pharmacist can ask, "do you take medicines for your hypertension"? or "do you apply anything externally for any skin infection"? Such questions make the patient recollect even the treatments that were given to them a long time back. Thus, prompting questions asked by pharmacists results in a fruitful interview. If the correct answer is not forthcoming even after prompting, the pharmacist has to rely on patients' family members or caretakers.

Interview Questions

Apart from the above, the pharmacists can ask questions regarding the new medicines given by the doctors, medicines stopped or changed over the course of time, etc. In order to get full information, the pharmacists can ask a number of questions on the use of OTC drugs mentioning the symptoms and diseases usually treated by the OTC drugs. Invariably, many chronic patients go to doctors of alternative systems of medicine, out of anxiety to get a cure for their longtime diseases. They try to hide any such treatments from the healthcare team owing to guilt or self-consciousness. They also hide their visits to many doctors of modern medicine at the same time. Only by winning the patient's faith and confidence, the pharmacists can dig out correct information. While questioning patients, the pharmacists should ask non-biased questions and avoid leading questions like, "you don't smoke, do you?" Leading questions prompt the patient with a particular answer.

Even pharmacists forget to ask some important questions during the interview. In order to avoid such lapses, the pharmacists can follow a certain pattern of asking questions such as a 24 hours survey and a review of systems of the human body. In the 24 hours survey pattern, questions can start from the patient's life of getting up from the bed in the morning to going to bed at night. Similarly, if questions are asked in alignment with the body system, diseases or treatment, a complete interview is possible.

Sometimes, even after so much pre-planning and organization, important information on medicines that are previously and currently used by the patient cannot be obtained. This could be owed to a single factor that the patient doesn't remember anything worth about their medicines. In such cases, the patient or their caregivers should be asked to bring all the medicines, even the empty containers. The patients should be educated to carry the list of the current medication, both the prescription and the OTC medicines. They should also be encouraged to stick to the same pharmacy by explaining all the benefits.

However, the information regarding the patient's non-compliance with instructions of doctors, pharmacists, and other healthcare team members is difficult to get. Nobody admits to their mistake easily. Hence, probing questions like the following should be asked to find out non-compliance:

1. Do you carry medicines to your workplace?

2. Do you forget some doses?

3. What will you do if you forget to refill the prescription?

4. If the medicine is inconvenient to you in any way, what will you do?

5. Do you use costly medicines as and when needed or as per doctor's instruction?

6. Have you ever increased or decreased the dose of a drug?

From the answers to these and similar other questions, non-compliance, drug misuse, and abuse can be guessed and such findings should be promptly intimated to the treating physician through the final report after medication history interview.

Essential Skills for Medication History Interview

Candace W Burnett, et al, has listed over 14 skills in the American Journal of Pharmaceutical Education [vol. 66, 2002] which are required for conducting a good medication history interview. They are given below:

1. The formal form of addressing the patient. [Good Morning Mr. X!]
2. Rapport with the patient. [Self-introduction, purpose, the time required]
3. Active listening, empathetic responding.
4. Open-ended questions
5. Closed-ended questions
6. The transition from one subject to another.[mention it for mental preparation]
7. Verbal involvement/ repeating the patient's own words.
8. Avoidance of leading questions
9. Avoidance of 'why' questions
10. Timing [giving time to adapt to a series of questions]
11. Clarifying conflicting information
12. Silence [allowing the patient to show emotion, digest information, etc.]
13. Answering questions by the patient
14. Mentioning the previous answer and question [to link current question]

If a clinical pharmacist develops the skills suggested above, a useful medication interview can be obtained. Thus, the quality of the information obtained from the patient and their caregivers depends on the quality of the pharmacist's interviewing and reviewing techniques, knowledge, and skills.

Closing an Interview

To close the interview, the pharmacist must highlight a part or maybe the entire interview with the patient. This permits the patient or the interviewer to correct any error, clear any confusion, confirm the information that is already given or add any new information. At the end of the interview, the pharmacist can ask for additional information which the patient think might be useful. Also, they can ask for the patient's opinions or reasons for the present problem. Additionally, one more opportunity can also be given to the patient to make corrections, if any. All these points should be noted in a short form during the interview and documented immediately after the interview as a report for the reference of the treating physician and the healthcare team.

Use of Patient's Case History in Evaluation of Drug Therapy

The evaluation of drug therapy or Drug Utilization Evaluation [DUE] is actually a quality improvement program by the hospital. The patient medication history, medication profile, and lab test profile are the three important documents that are necessary to carry out DUE. Among the three, the medication history plays an important role. It is used as the starting point to commence the treatment. Hence, the other members of the healthcare team like doctors, nurses, and lab technologists also ask the patient a few questions to get proper medication history. They also record it in the documents that they prepare. There may be discrepancies or conflicts of information in the histories noted by the pharmacists and others. Such aberrations should be discussed with the staff concerned and the necessary corrections should be made after a proper clarification with the patient.

As all this information is evaluated and compared during DUE, it is important to present correct and reliable data to the DUE committee. These data help the DUE committee to identify

1. Medication error, either during the present or a previous therapy
2. Untreated indications or undetected illness
3. The correctness of present therapy
4. Any improvement required in present drug use

Above all, the DUE team appreciates the usefulness of medication history.

Thus, patient medication history not only helps to commence the treatment but also to conclude it with DUE.

QUESTIONS

1. Explain briefly the difference between patient medication interview and counseling.
2. How should one prepare for conducting a medication history interview?
3. Write a note on the structure of the patient's case history.

4. How is the patient's case history useful in DUE?
5. List the skills required for conducting Medication History Interview
6. What are the advantages of a Medication History Interview?
7. How do you conduct a medication history interview?
8. Explain the role of body language while conducting medication history interview.
9. List different types of questions with examples and discuss their importance.
10. Conduct a mock medication history interview with one of your classmates as patient and submit a report on the same.

C H A P T E R **10**

COMMUNITY PHARMACY MANAGEMENT

LEARNING OBJECTIVE

The chapter provides some ideas about managing a community pharmacy. Important sections of management science like finance management, materials management, and human resources management are explained which on learning a reader can use while practicing the profession.

WHAT IS MANAGEMENT?

Management is an art as well as the science of planning, organizing, directing, and controlling efforts and resources of an organization. The basis of management is decision making. After identifying and defining a problem, it is analyzed, different solutions are found and the best solution is implemented by the management. A long time ago, the management and administration of a firm were considered one and the same but now it has been established that the former is concerned with decision making and the latter has more to do with implementation. However, this is not a fixed rule as there is a considerable amount of overlapping in the functions of these two.

COMMUNITY PHARMACY MANAGEMENT

As far as the community pharmacy management is concerned, it is about the functioning of a small organization. However, even they have to follow the basic principles of management. They have to deal with men, material and finance alike. Thus, there are three categories for the same:

1. Financial management

2.   Materials [infrastructure] management and

3.   Human resources [staff] management.

1. FINANCIAL MANAGEMENT

The very first requirement to run a pharmacy is capital. In order to estimate the amount of capital required, the following three points are taken into consideration.

1. Estimated or expected sales volume

2. Inventory required to meet the above and

3. Approximate operating expenses

All the above three are estimated by thorough research, market survey, and from the experience of the people of the locality. Usually, the projected sales volume is estimated at a lower level while the operating expenses are estimated at a higher level so as to avoid any kind of disappointment. In the initial stages, the capital requirements will be more as the suppliers or wholesalers may not be forthcoming to offer credit. However, it may change favorably in the due course of time. Similarly, if the pharmacy desires to go for credit sale to the customers, the capital requirement increases.

Capital is required to pay advance rent for the building, creating infrastructure inside the pharmacy, and more importantly, for purchasing inventory and stock, whereas, cash is required to meet the operating expenses and for emergency purchases and expenses. As much as possible, fixtures and equipment are fixed and installed in the manner that they are movable and relocated if required. This minimizes the waste and helps in the recovery of capital.

Financial management also includes efficient management of money or cash in the business. This is reflected in the return on the investment. Generally, the cash flow in a business is limited but the demand usually exceeds the supply. In these circumstances, efficiency in finance/money management is of utmost importance. In case of a failure, the pharmacy will not be able to honor its payment commitment to suppliers and will lose all the potential discounts on cash purchases.

2. MATERIALS/INFRASTRUCTURE MANAGEMENT

The objective of materials management is its continuous flow to the pharmacy without any interruption. Hence, controlling the inventory of a pharmacy acquires significance. It is further described in detail in Chapter No. 19. Inventory control is more important for a pharmacy because of its limited resources. A peculiar problem that arises with the community pharmacy is that there is no way to estimate the demand and quantify it precisely or even approximately. This is because the demand for a prescription is generated by physicians and not by the consumers. Dealing with the consumer for product requirements is easier as compared to having to deal with the doctors. For example, if a particular general item stock has accumulated and is in excess, it can be pushed to consumers by offering discounts, incentives, etc. On the other hand, it is not possible in the case of drugs. Hence, a very careful inventory level has to be managed so as to avoid excess or shortage. Another problem with drugs is its immediate need as the patient cannot be requested to wait till we procure and supply it the next day or later. While maintaining stock of a particular drug, the prescription flow, its frequency and the time taken by the vendors to deliver must be taken into account.

CONTROL ON PURCHASES

Having said all this regarding the control on purchases, a community pharmacist should not be too strict on purchases because once they earn the reputation of 'out of stock pharmacy", they will lose patrons in no time.

INFRASTRUCTURE REQUIREMENT AND ITS MANAGEMENT

The infrastructure includes fixtures and equipment for proper storage, display, and sale. For a community pharmacy, apart from the legal requirement of the refrigerator, air conditioner, storage racks, dispensing counter, etc, computer, printer, arrangement for uninterrupted power supply is a major requirement. For taking care of the above-mentioned factors, multiple quotations can be collected and the best supplier can be picked for hassle-free operations. In order to fix the infrastructures, proper consultations with experts is a must. After considering an increase in sales volume, convenience of employees, customers, ambiance, and appearance, the layout of the pharmacy should be decided.

The modern fixtures are designed to offer flexibility and it is important to experiment with them against various arrangements and layouts until a most suitable combination is achieved.

3. HUMAN RESOURCE [STAFF] MANAGEMENT

Depending upon the size of the community pharmacy, there could be a requirement of one cashier cum accountant, two or more pharmacy assistants or salesmen. This is independent of the legal requirement of a full-time pharmacist. If the pharmacy is open for more than 8 hours in a day, an even bigger staff may be required. Most of the pharmacies operate from 9 am to 9 pm without interval. Hence, there must be at least 2 sets of employees. As most of the patients prefer visiting either early morning or after 5 pm, a skeleton staff during the day time and a wider staff during evening hours can be one ideal pattern for human resource management. If the pharmacy decides to serve the community round the clock, additional staff may be required during the night shift.

The pharmacy assistants selected for the job should have some prior experience in community pharmacy. If not, they should be properly trained in the day to day operations and also made aware of neat housekeeping. Their services should be used to arrange and display the goods received. They can also help clean the racks periodically and verify the drugs for expiry date, damage, leakage, etc. also while cleaning them individually and replacing the dead ones. This helps in avoiding the unexpected loss due to the expiry of stocks to a larger extent. For similar reasons, new arrivals should be kept behind the old stock. However, this is not a concrete rule as sometimes the drugs with short expiry might be supplied later. If the community pharmacy opts for door delivery of drugs to the customer, at least one assistant with a two-wheeler driving license should be recruited.

As the pharmacists have to concentrate on patient-oriented services like patient counseling, noting medication history, giving instructions about the use of drugs, clarifying patients' doubts, placing orders, receiving medical representatives, etc., the pharmacy assistants can be trained to maintain the stock of non-medical products like baby food, cosmetics, and other general items. This way, they get to develop a rapport with regular customers and also get a better sense of the business.

Thus human resource management is an important aspect of community pharmacy management which has the potential of making or breaking a pharmacy.

QUESTIONS

1. What is management?

2. Briefly explain the financial management of a community pharmacy

3. Write a note on Materials management in a community pharmacy

4. Explain Staff Management of a community pharmacy

5. Write about the management of a community pharmacy in detail.

CHAPTER 11

PHARMACY AND THERAPUETICS COMMITTEE

LEARNING OBJECTIVE

The objectives are to paint a complete picture of one of the valuable committees of a hospital. The organization and functions of the committee are explained in detail. Particularly the functions of PTC in each and every problem encountered in a hospital are analyzed under separate headings. Thus by learning the chapter the student upon graduation, should able to appreciate the committee's works and able to serve better in it, if a chance is given.

INTRODUCTION

In the last few decades, spurt in the field of scientific knowledge and the availability of advanced electronic equipment has lead to the introduction of thousands of new drugs in the market. According to an estimate, there are more than 70,000 formulations available in India for prescribing by doctors. Now, it is impossible to remember these many formulations along with their uses and merits. Hence, it becomes necessary that the hospital establishes a system to bring the best medicine to the attention of the staff and this assists them in the proper selection of drugs for the treatment of patients. This educational programme is achieved through 'Pharmacy and Therapeutic Committee' formed in the hospitals.

It is a committee of the medical and paramedical staff that serves as a liaison between the medical staff and the pharmacy service on all matters pertaining to the use of drugs in the hospital.

DEFINITION

Hassan defines Pharmacy and Therapeutic Committee as *"a policy framing and recommending body to the medical staff and the administration of the hospital on matters related to the safe and rational use of drugs"*.

OBJECTIVES

There are three major roles of the Pharmacy and Therapeutics Committee:

1. Advisory
2. Education and
3. Safe and rational use of drugs

1. Advisory

As mentioned earlier, the primary role of the PTC is to assist the physician in the proper selection of drugs. The PTC advises on the formulation and adaptation of policies regarding evolution, selection and therapeutic use of drugs in hospitals. To sum up, its main objective is to serve in an advisory capacity to the medical staff and hospital administration in all matters related to the use of drugs including investigational drugs. Furthermore, it also advises the pharmacy department regarding effective drug distribution and control.

2. Education

PTC helps the administration of hospitals in formulating programs to meet the educational needs of all the staff concerned like Physicians, Nurses, Pharmacists, and other health care professionals to update their knowledge on the matters related to drugs and their use. Towards this objective, PTC is entrusted with the responsibility of selecting staff for continuing education program and also preparing and updating of Hospital formulary – a valuable reference book for hospital staff.

3. Safe and rational use of drugs

As the medicines today are highly potent and powerful, one has to take extra care while handling, administering, and using the drugs. The correct use of the drugs can be ensured upon following the PTC's standard instructions. However, in reality, the medical staff, nurses and pharmacists usually overlook these guidelines, resulting in irrational and dangerous use of drugs. When an adverse incident involving the use of drugs happens and gets reported, no one is ready to take the blame. In order to avoid a situation like this, the PTC repeatedly warns the staff not to ignore its guidelines on matters pertaining to the safe and rational use of drugs. Thus, the first two objectives of advice and education are to achieve the final objective of the safe use of drugs.

ORGANIZATION

The organization of the committee may vary from hospital to hospital. However, the following composition is followed in general:

1. A minimum of 3 physicians from among the medical staff of the hospital.

2. A Pharmacist (usually the HOD or chief pharmacist)

3. A Nurse and

4. An Administrator

One among the above physicians is appointed as the chairman of the committee. The pharmacist is designated as the secretary.

PTC also constitutes several sub-committees, which are either permanent or formed for a specific purpose temporarily. In these sub-committees, specialists are included either as president or members in order to utilize their knowledge and experience in the particular field. There may be a sub-committee on Antibiotics, cardiovascular drugs, hormones and corticosteroids, narcotics, and other CNS drugs.

PTC can also invite people from within or outside the hospital to its meetings who can contribute their specialized knowledge and judgments on the matters of interest. The committee must meet regularly at least six times a year or more, if necessary. Like any standard committee, the secretary should keep track of the timing of the meeting with all the other necessary documents. The decisions of the committee are communicated to the people concerned and executed by the secretary. The secretary also reports these tasks to the committee members in the next meeting of the committee.

Primary Functions

Though PTC has advisory and educational objectives, the primary aim of the PTC is the safe and rational use of drugs in the hospital. In order to achieve that objective, PTC plays an important role in:

1. Adverse Drug Reaction (ADR) monitoring

2. Drug product defect reporting

3. Psychotropic drugs use

4. Emergency drugs use

5. Drug utilization review and

6. Safe use of all drugs

Each of the above functions is meticulously carried out by PTC by issuing necessary regulations and guidelines to the staff concerned. Let us have a look at these guidelines in detail.

1. **Adverse drug reaction monitoring (PTC and ADR):** Adverse drug reaction is defined as a reaction that is noxious, unintended, and occurs at normal doses used for humans. Though it occurs less frequently, the cause for it must be thoroughly investigated to prevent such reactions in other patients or at least to be vigilant on all patients given the drug in question.

In order to do so, some organizations in the hospital must be given charge of this responsibility. PTC takes up this responsibility and monitors the therapy throughout the hospital. Its main aim is to prevent ADR and if occurred, to take follow-up actions that include treatment of the particular patient, reporting to authorities concerned, and avoids such ADR in the future.

For doing it effectively, PTC issues a set of guidelines to the medical and Para-medical staff of the hospital including an ADR reporting form to report the incident. The model ADR reporting form is given below:

Name of the Hospital and Location

Adverse Drug Reaction Report

Ref. No: Date: ....

Patient's Name:

Age/sex:

Hospital O.P/I.P/Regn. No.:

Disease reported/diagnosed

Details of treatment given:

Drug suspected to have produced ADR:

Detail about that drug (B. No, Mfg. Date, Exp. date, Manufacturer's Address):

Reaction Detail:

Step taken to treat ADR:

Drug in question prescribed by:

Administered by:

Other drugs concurrently administered or taken by patient, if any:

Any other relevant information:

Department/   *Signature of treating*

Ward   *physician with date*

N.B: The packing or container or balance of the suspected drugs should be retained for further reference and investigation.

Upon receiving ADR report from the concerned department or ward, PTC starts its investigation to find out the cause for that particular ADR. If necessary, it calls for further information from the reporting physician, nurse or even the patient. At the end of an investigation by its sub-committee, specially assigned this duty, PTC submits its report to the concerned authorities. Usually, it is reported first to the Dean or Director of the hospital and then to ADR reporting authority of the State or Central Government and then to State Drugs Control Authorities. Depending upon the seriousness and frequency of this ADR, the drug in question may be withdrawn from the market on the orders of Drugs Control Department. They can also issue a strict warning to the medical fraternity to be vigilant while using the particular drug through press and mass media.

2. **Drug product defect reporting (PTC and drug's defect):** Generally, everybody involved in the usage of a particular drug, especially patients and the doctors expect a zero error or 100% defect free product. However, this is not always possible. Owing to factors like machine errors or human errors, the drug reaches the user point with some or the other noticeable defects. However, these defects should be detected by the pharmacist, nurse, or doctor before it reaches to the patient. If detected, they are duty-bound to report the same to the PTC of the hospital.

Reportable defects include inadequate packing, confusing or inadequate labels, deteriorated, contaminated dosage forms, inaccurate fill, faulty drug delivering apparatus, etc. The health care professionals should report anything which, in their professional opinion is considered to be defective or undesirably associated with the drug product.

The model form for reporting the defective drug product is given below:

PTC, on receiving the above report initiates an investigation and takes possession of the suspected drug product from the reporter. After verification, it reports the matter to the manufacturer and then to the other authorities concerned, if required. It further orders a physical inspection of the entire lot of the product supplied to the hospital and takes necessary action.

By this program, a sense of vigilance and duty consciousness is instilled in the minds of health care professionals that help in delivering defect free products to the patients.

3. **Psychotropic drugs use (PTC and dangerous drugs):** Psychotropic drugs are those which create dependence or addiction on longer use. This is dangerous to the patient and the society alike. Hence, they are also termed as dangerous drugs. PTC develops guidelines whereby dangerous drugs are purchased, stored, dispensed, and properly administered under control.

The procedure for this is similar to the Psychotropic Substances Acts and rules. The PTC ensures strict adherence to the above Act by the hospital staff. In some hospitals, automatic stop orders are enforced whereby "all drug orders for narcotics, sedatives, and hypnotics shall be automatically discontinued after 48 hours, unless

1. the order indicates the exact number of doses to be given

2. an exact period of time for the medication is specified and

3. the attending physician records the medication."

In some other hospitals, the automatic stop orders require, "all orders for narcotics, sedatives, and hypnotics must be rewritten every 24 hours". Thus, the PTC takes care of the use of psychotropic drugs and the patients of the hospital.

NAME OF THE HOSPITAL

ADDRESS

DRUGS DEFECT REPORT

REF.NO.   DATE:

1. Name of the drug:

2. Dosage form and strength:

3. Batch No. ------ Dt. of Mfg ----- Expiry Date:----------

4. Manufacturer's Name and Address:

5. Date of purchase:

6. Name of the supplier and address:

7. Defects noted or suspected:

8. Reported by (Name and Designation)

9. Signature

10. Department/ward

N.B: The suspected defective drug should be preserved for further investigation.

4. Emergency drugs use (PTC and emergency drugs): As time factor is very important during emergency cases, the PTC prepares a list of drugs and other supplies to be made available in emergency boxes. These boxes are kept in all important places of the hospital within the charge of a pharmacist or nursing supervisors of the hospital.

As these medicines are literally available by the side of the beds of the emergency cases, they are referred to as 'Bedside Pharmacy'.

After the emergency cupboards have been placed on the wards and other places like emergency procedures room of the department of radiology, it is mandatory that a program is developed where these drugs are checked daily, either by the hospital pharmacist or by the nursing supervisor responsible for the ward. The drug used on the day is replenished, as early as possible, so that a constant amount of drugs are always available in the emergency cupboard.

Usually, the emergency boxes have over 30 items of important, life-saving drugs and about 10 to 15 items of surgical instruments and dressings including syringes and needles. The list may vary depending upon the need of a particular hospital which may decide to add or delete some items in the emergency boxes. Overall, the PTC of the hospital is responsible for the preparation and up-keeping of the emergency Drugs kit or 'Bedside Pharmacy'.

The following list of content is given to serve as a guide

Emergency Drugs

1. Aminophylline 0.25 gm/10ml
2. Amphetamine sulphate 20mg/ml
3. Amyl nitrite inhalation
4. Atropine sulphate 0.4mg/ml
5. Caffeine sodium benzoate 0.5 gm/2ml
6. Calcium gluconate 1 gm/10ml
7. Chlorpheniramine maleate 10 mg/ml
8. Digoxin 0.25mg/ml
9. Diphenylhydantoin sodium 50mg/ml
10. Epinephrine Hydrochloride 1:1000
11. Heparin 10,000units/ml
12. Hydrocortisone 100mg
13. Isoproterenol1:100
14. Magnesium sulphate injection 10% and50%
15. Mannitol injection25%
16. NalorphineHCl 10 mg/2ml
17. Neostigmine Methylsulphate 0.25 mg/ml
18. Nor. epinephrine Injection0.2%
19. Pentobarbital 50mg/ml
20. Phenobarbital 120mg/ml
21. Phenylephrine HCl 10mg/ml
22. Picrotoxin injection 3mg/ml
23. Procainamide 100mg/ml
24. Protamine sulphate 10mg/ml
25. Saline for injection 30ml
26. Sodium molar Lactate solution
27. Water for injection 50ml

Other Items

1. Syringes of all sizes – each2
2. Needles of all sizes – each 2
3. Venous cannulatization set
4. Oxygen catheters
5. Sterile suction catheters

6. Razor with blades

7. Sterile gelatin sponge

8. Resuscitation tube & cart

9. Oxygen equipment

10. Burn sheets and

11. Other surgical instruments like scissors, forceps, etc.

5. **Drug utilization review: (PTC and drugs use):** Drug utilization includes prescribing, dispensing, and administering of the prescription drugs. Though there is no drug utilization review outside a hospital, such a review can be organized in a hospital by PTC. Providing "Hospital formulary" is one of the institutional methods to control the drug utilization as well as a mechanism for continuing education of physicians, nurses, and pharmacists. There are some policies framed by PTC for including or excluding a drug in hospital formulary. They are further discussed in the chapter on "Hospital Formulary". Similarly, the PTC also circulates policies on inpatient and outpatient prescriptions which describe the quantity duration, antibiotic use, etc.

Obtaining 'Medication History' of the patient and maintaining 'patient medication profile' are the other two programs that are useful for a pharmacist to monitor drug utilization within the hospital.

The medication histories of required patients admitted to the hospital or in the outpatient department are noted by the clinical pharmacist. This is either accomplished by personal interview or through a computerized questionnaire specifically designed for the purpose and if the patient is in a condition to answer those questions. If not, the interview is conducted at an appropriate time but at the earliest, with the help of patient's helpers or family members. During the interview, details regarding medicines taken recently, at the time of admission and OTC drugs used are collected.

Additionally, important information regarding the known drug allergies, idiosyncrasy towards food products and lab tests involving anything that is conducted using diagnostic agents is also recorded. This information is passed on to the treating physician for early diagnosis and prescribing.

Once this is over, the patient's medication profile is prepared in the following format:

NAME OF THE HOSPITAL

ADDRESS

PATIENT MEDICATION PROFILE

No: Date:

Patient's Name

Age/sex

Address

Hospital OP/IP Regn. No.

Date of Admission

Diagnosis on Admission

Other pathology

Drug Profile

Date	Name of the Drug	Dose	Route	Started on	Stopped on	Remark	Ph. initial

Discharged on:

Signature of Chief Pharmacist

The patient medication profile can be prepared and maintained by both the hospital pharmacists and the community pharmacists because drug utilization review is not possible without the medication history of the patient. The community pharmacists can maintain patient medication profile of those who frequently visit the pharmacies for procuring medicines for themselves and their family members. Their services are very useful in the case of patients requiring long time therapy and those who continue treatment from their homes as outpatients for diseases like diabetes, hypertension, asthma, epilepsy and TB.

Modern community pharmacies that employ graduate pharmacists and have proper computer systems are offering such services to the patients.

6. **PTC and safe use of drugs:** Everyday, a lot of new drugs are introduced by hundreds of pharmaceutical manufacturers throughout the world. Consequently, the responsibilities of health care professionals, pharmacists in particular, also increase many folds. The possibilities of error in prescription writing, dispensing and administration of these new drugs poses a great problem to the pharmacist, especially when the chances for Drug interaction, ADR, and other problems are relatively unknown for the new drugs.

Hence, the PTC formulates several policies and guidelines to be followed by everyone concerned while handling new and existing drugs. The following are some of the guidelines:

1. The hospital should appoint a qualified pharmacist to supervise the entire pharmacy services. They must be a graduate in pharmacy with adequate experience.

2. All dispensing operations must be carried out by qualified registered pharmacists. Non-pharmacy people should not be engaged for dispensing.

3. An adequate number of pharmacists must be appointed, proportionate to the workload and round the clock service.

4. The hospital must provide adequate and safe workspace and storage facilities for the pharmacy.

5. The hospital should have a hospital formulary and it should be updated regularly or at least once in a year.

6. The pharmacist must follow all the rules regarding the storage and dispensing of narcotics, poison, and external use preparations.

7. In the hospital manufacturing section, the drugs should be manufactured according to Current Good Manufacturing Practice (CGMP) and other rules by the Drugs Control Department. Furthermore, strict quality control and quality assurance measures must be followed.

8. All wards and nursing stations should be periodically checked for expired drugs, deteriorated drugs, legibility of labels, etc.

9. The pharmacy should have a small library with reference books on pharmacology, toxicology, posology and pharmacopeia, hospital formulary, drug index, etc and

10. Periodical continuing education programs should be conducted by the hospital for the staff and attendance for those programs must be compulsory.

Following these PTC guidelines in letter and spirit can ensure safe use of drugs in the hospitals.

Other Functions of PTC

1. The manufacturing unit of the hospital is inspected by the PTC for quality production.

2. The PTC also visits outside manufacturing units before approving their products for inclusion in hospital formulary or purchase lists.

3. It prepares written policies and procedures for the evaluation, selection, purchase, storage, dispensing, and usage of drugs. It also prepares guidelines for the inpatient and outpatient prescriptions along with an automatic stop order.

4. It prepares the Hospital formulary while also updating it periodically. It also documents the policies for including drugs into formulary which is discussed in the chapter on Hospital Formulary.

5. It forms sub-committees on the essential subjects and

6. It establishes procedures for cost-effective drug therapy.

QUESTIONS

1. Define PTC.

2. What are the objectives of PTC?

3. Who are the members PTC?

4. Write a note on PTC and emergency drugs.

5. What are the functions of PTC?

6. Elaborate the functions of PTC.

7. Explain the role of PTC in the safe use of drugs.

8. Justify the need for forming PTC in hospitals.

9. How PTC controls ADR in hospitals?

CHAPTER 12

DRUG INFORMATION SERVICES AND POISON INFORMATION CENTRE

LEARNING OBJECTIVE

Upon completion of the chapter, a student should be able to establish, maintain and function in a DIC or PIC. Since the very important aspect of such centers is the availability of a large number of information resources, they are elaborately dealt with in this chapter. Thus the chapter aims to make the student the best receiver and provider of information from these centers.

INTRODUCTION

Traditionally, the pharmacists only provided limited information about drugs like dosage, use, and storage to the patients visiting hospitals and retail outlets. This process has now changed from product-oriented to patient-oriented. They are now expected to provide all information regarding drugs along with other related information like availability, substitute, ADR, research findings, etc. To help with this, drug information centers are established in all the big hospitals and other places. As the custodian of knowledge bank (Drug Information Centre, DIC), a pharmacist is expected to play a much larger role as a teacher and information provider.

Need for Drug Information Centers

Owing to rapid scientific developments and consequent research possibilities in the last few decades, a lot of new drugs and formulations are added to the book of drugs every day throughout the world. Now, the volume of information available about drugs is impossible to manage by an individual, irrespective of their experience and education. Therefore, there is a need for an efficient management system to collect, edit and arrange such a huge quantity of information. This makes the drug information centers an essential entity.

Moreover, all the published information is not needed by everybody. For example, for a cancer hospital, the information related to its activities is essential while the rest of the information is only of academic interest. So, there is a need for someone who could collect and edit the required information and bring it to their attention. This also becomes an overwhelming task due to a large number of journals and magazines in each subdivision of science nowadays. With the revolution in the information technology sector, there is information overflow from all around the world and hence, the need for dedicated service to sort out the required information. That brings the Drug Information services in the picture.

A busy practicing physician or surgeon is often in need of urgent information during a complicated situation. In order to procure that information, they will be investing a lot of energy and time. However, if a center or service is available for ready reference, it will save them the trouble. Moreover, even the general public can reach out to Drug Information centers to clarify their doubts regarding the drugs they use or the diseases without much effort and money. The lack of such centers increases their dependence on the treating physician. Most of the time, people are reluctant and, in turn, deprived of the essential information. This might result in severe complications.

Thus, the need for Drug Information Centre is evident.

Suitable Person to be in charge of DIC

In a hospital setup, the pharmacist is a member of the Pharmacy and Therapeutic Committee, and in charge of the hospital library. So, that poses a strong candidature for them being in charge of the Drug Information Centre.

Usually, the information is provided by drug manufacturers, distributors, and their representatives. By nature of their job, the pharmacist is always in touch with these sources of information. They can collect those details easily. Also, these information suppliers are fellow pharmacists, employees, making the process easier.

Pharmacists undergo a thorough education about drugs and their physical, chemical, pharmaceutical, and pharmacological properties for a few years. They are more knowledgeable than others about drugs which is useful in critically evaluating all literature available about the drugs and selecting the correct information. This information can be edited by them and passed on to whoever needs it. It is safe to conclude that a pharmacist is the most suitable candidate to be in charge of the Drug Information Centre.

Establishing D.I.C

To establish a DIC, a pharmacist must pay attention to three important aspects. The first and foremost is information gathering and storing. The second one is information retrieval, and the last one is information dissemination.

For information gathering, the following sources of information should be approached and the relevant materials purchased. Textbooks, journals, and other printed materials from different publishers can be of great help. Apart from these printed hard copies, there are database soft copies that can be purchased from the authorities and the suppliers concerned. Their price range varies from a few thousand rupees to a few lakh rupees per copy.

Moreover, all Drug Information Centres should have an ideal internet connection with high download speed. In order to supplement the information thus collected, literature and booklets published by pharmaceutical manufacturers, National Pharmaceutical, and Medical associations should be collected and kept ready for reference. Nowadays, all the Drug Information Centres and libraries of Universities of Health Sciences and colleges are networked. So, it is easier to collect information from any of these institutions.

For information retrieval, the DIC pharmacist should establish and maintain a system for quick retrieval from the available sources. The retrieval of the information from internet sources is explained in detail later in this chapter. However, reference books hard copies, pharmacopeias, and journals are equally important for information retrieval. The DIC should have a bucca catalog of these books arranged according to the topics, subjects, publishers, authors, much like a public library. This can be done using software that should be installed in DIC computers. While the available information can be retrieved quickly, there is always a fair chance that it is insufficient and questionable.

The unavailable information can be gathered from other sources in the network which may require a little more time. As most of the information sought from DIC may be for immediate adaptation and implementation, the pharmacist should get the information as quickly as possible. However, the information or data of doubtful nature requires clarification. Those details have to be passed on to a panel of drug consultants. After seeking their opinion on the same, this information can be provided to the seeker. Hence, DIC needs to constitute a panel of pharmacy experts. Sometimes, the DIC pharmacists themselves have to critically evaluate the drug information and literature before adding them to the collections.

The third important aspect of DIC is the dissemination of information. This requires a systematic approach.

Sources of Information

Based on the origin and nature of the information the sources of information can be divided into three. They are:

1. Primary sources
2. Secondary sources and
3. Tertiary sources

1. **Primary Sources:** These are the original information generated by research scholars and scientists, and are published either in scientific journals or presented in conferences, seminars. This information is not condensed, interpreted, or edited by a second party. Other examples are patent applications, theses, dissertations, and technical reports.

2. **Secondary Sources:** This information is collected from all or any one of the above primary sources. It is edited and interpreted by people other than the original authors. Usually, it is done for a specific purpose, catering to a particular audience. These include review articles, handbooks, textbooks, encyclopedias, and computerized services like abstracting or indexing services. Read on for a detailed description on this.

3. Tertiary Sources: The information derived from both or either of the above sources is known as Tertiary information. Here, the information provided is composite and in a diluted version. Examples are guides, pamphlets issued by manufacturers. The information gathered from people who attended the conferences and seminars also comes under this category.

We can now conclude that the primary sources of information are reliable, accurate, and recently updated. On the other hand, the secondary and tertiary information sources are less accurate because they travel through several authors and publishers.

Computerized Services

This is one of the secondary sources of information where details are collected from various sources, edited and published as databases in CD.ROM format or uploaded on internet websites and portals. They are further differentiated into indexing services and abstracting services. Both these services are quite useful for libraries and information centers like Drug Information centers. Here, a simple online search can be used for browsing through the database of remote locations with no network facilities. On the other hand, a CD can be useful when a lot of people are using the same machine.

Abstracting Services: As the name indicates, it contains the summaries and abstracts of original reports. It also interprets the original report according to the editorial guidelines. Popular examples are:

(a)　Drugdex

(b)　International Pharmaceutical Abstract

(c)　Pharmline

Pharmline database (http://www.pharmline.com) is an abstracting system that deals with drugs and professional pharmacy practice. This database abstracts articles on pharmacy practice and clinical use of drugs from over 100 English pharmacy and medical journals produced by National Health Service Information specialists.

International pharmaceutical abstracts are produced by the American Society of Health System (ASHP) pharmacists. It contains articles published in more than 750 pharmacies, medical and other health-related journals, published worldwide. This service started in the year 1970. It is a paid service, available via http://www.ashp.org/ipal.

Indexing Services

Following are the examples of indexing services:

1. Medline

2. BIOSIS [Biosciences information service] previews

3. Clinalert

4. Embase and

5. IDIS (Iowa drug Information System)

Indexing service is not interpreting the original article but providing only the indexed topic and the original abstract or full text.

1. **Medline:** In this indexing service, medical, dental, and nursing journals are indexed which is prepared by the US National Library of Medicine. Since 1966, over 11 million records from more than 4300 journals have been indexed in this service. However, "The Pharmaceutical Journal" is not covered in this one. This database is updated daily and its CD versions like OVID and silver platter are easily available. The Medline system via the internet includes 'Pubmed' and 'Biomed net'. They only differ in their presentation and search systems.

2. **BIOSIS:** [Biosciences information service] It has a collection of journals, meetings, books, and patent data that we need to prepare research projects, grant proposals, and follow trends in the life sciences. BIOSIS research databases provide us with the current sources of life sciences information including journals, conferences, patents, books, review articles and more.

3. **Clinalert:** It contains the comprehensive summaries of adverse drug reactions, drug interactions and market withdrawals from over 100 key medical and research journals from around the world.

4. **Embase:** This is published by Elsevier Science. It is a major database covering pharmaceutical and biomedical journals. It contains more than 4000 indexed international journals and over 8 million records from 1974.

5. **Iowa Drug Information Service (IDIS):** It is published by the University of Iowa, USA. It covers about 200 important English medical and pharmaceutical journals. This one contains the articles relating to human treatment, available in their full version. It is available on both the internet and a CD ROM.

Retrieval of Information

Since a database contains a lot of information, retrieval requires skills. If you are looking for the correct terms, the retrieval becomes easier. In order to do that, use the indexing language of the database (controlled vocabulary or thesaurus or keywords). One can use all the possible synonyms to make the search easier. On the contrary, the use of common language and free text will not help in retrieving all the relevant information. So, before starting the search, a clear question must be framed. For example, "How effective are ACE inhibitors in the treatment of heart failure?" The next step is to choose relevant subject headings and keywords to include in the search. These can be included in the search question using the Boolean operators (and/or/not) to get relevant citations. Some databases like Medline and Embase use subheadings like Adverse effects, Use, Diagnosis, etc, to direct the search towards the specific question.

POISON INFORMATION CENTRE [PIC]

Importance of PIC

Intentional or accidental, poisoning can occur at any time. It can be fatal if not treated immediately. Hence, the required information is always urgent. Usually, the inquiries are made through phone and a quick reply is expected at the moment. As it is a matter of life and death, Poison Information Centres must be open round the clock throughout the year. Thus, it differs from the Drug Information Centre where the inquiries are not always urgent except for some rare occasions.

Sources of Poison

There can be various sources of poison ranging from natural sources to synthetic sources. The natural sources include plants, animals, and minerals whereas the synthetic sources are cosmetics, household items, and pharmaceuticals. Most of the time, the chemicals including drugs act as poisons. These chemicals can be obtained from agricultural or horticultural sources. Rarely laboratory chemicals cause poison. The next major source of poison common to the majority of the Indian population is poisonous plants of wild growth. Fungi, cosmetics, and household items like disinfectants, acids, and even diamonds are used to commit suicide. Small children can accidentally swallow anything that comes to their hands. Thus, the sources of poison are vast and unimaginable.

Information about Poisons

In order to treat the poison cases effectively and immediately, all the information about the said poison must be available. Hence, the data should be collected beforehand and kept ready. However, in practice, there are a number of problems in treating poison cases. Most of the time, the substances responsible for the poisoning is unknown because the patient might not be in a position to reveal it. The people accompanying the patients must bring the container, box, tube or paper found near the patient to the treating hospital. This could be of great help in poison identification. The next step is to estimate the quantity of poison consumed by the patient, which can only be guessed.

This is followed by checking the composition of the product consumed. The composition is labeled for the drugs and formulations while for other industrial products, it remains unknown. Hence, the least we could do is gather the information regarding the commonly used poisons from manufacturers and stock antidotes for using in emergency situations. Even after this, there are complications like the unknown properties of the finished product as the manufacturers can only reveal raw materials. Sometimes, the manufacturers are reluctant to disclose their secret formula. But when compelled by law for the purpose of treating poisons, they reveal it and that should be kept confidential. In a few instances, manufacturers change the composition without declaring it in labels. Thus, the treatment of poison cases is very difficult and most of the time, only symptomatic treatment is given.

However, a poison information center should collect the poison information as much as possible from as many sources as they can. The usual reference books available are:

1. Chemical toxicology of commercial products – By Gleason, et al.
2. Treatment of common acute poisoning – clinical – By Mathew. H. et al.
3. Hand Book of poisoning – By Driesbach
4. Extra pharmacopeia and
5. Merck Index etc.

Storage of Information

The information collected by these centers should be arranged in such a way that it is easier to retrieve. Earlier, the data were arranged alphabetically in written cards and handled manually.

Nowadays, this job is done by computers and the information can be retrieved in a fraction of the second. In order to have as much information as possible about each poison, the following format can be followed:

1. Name of the poison
2. Synonym
3. Source: Synthetic / plant / animal / mineral
4. Family (In case of plant or animal poison)
5. Description of external characters (macroscopy)
6. Habitat
7. Minimum lethal dose
8. Toxic effects
9. Symptoms
10. Pharmacokinetic properties
11. Treatment including antidotes
12. Supportive therapy
13. Prognosis
14. Any other relevant points and
15. References

Providing Information

This is not a mechanical job to be carried out by any non-health care professionals. It requires expertise to provide the needed information with all professional details in the shortest possible time. In order to do so, one needs to have an understanding of the basic principles of poison treatment. So, a pharmacist must gather that knowledge also from relevant sources.

Depending upon the time and weather first aid has been given to the patient, the required information varies. So, it is important to clarify these details first. The professional and clinical information is required for doctors, nurses and other health care professionals, but the people, in general, should also know about the first aid and what to do next. They should be advised accordingly and then instructed to contact later after visiting a nearby hospital or clinic. The remaining information can be shared during the second call.

As far as possible, detailed information should be given directly to the doctor. All these conversations depend on pharmacist's discretion and skill. The details of each inquiry should be properly recorded in the registers.

Follow up: The job of the Drug Information Centre pharmacist does not end after providing the information in the poison cases. They have to follow it up and obtain relevant details from the treating physician, nurses and relatives of the patient. These details may be useful for future cases and are appreciated by physicians.

QUESTIONS

1. Write briefly about the need for the Drug Information Centre.

2. How is a pharmacist suitable to manage DIC?

3. What are the sources of Drug Information?

4. List the function of the Drug Information Centre.

5. Write briefly about the importance of PIC.

6. Write in detail about the secondary source of information including the computerized sources.

7. Explain how the information about poison is provided in a poison information center.

8. How is a Drug Information Centre established?

CHAPTER 13

PATIENT COUNSELING

LEARNING OBJECTIVE

The chapter dealt with the following aspects: Definition, Need for Counseling, Classification, Special cases that require counseling, Preparation for counseling, Scope of counseling, Effect or uses of Counseling and Barriers or Problems in Patient Counseling. Thus it aims at providing near-complete information about the topic and hence the student should be able to adapt it while in pharmacy practice. That is the objective of learning the chapter.

DEFINITION

Patient counseling is a form of patient education as the majority of information provided during counseling is for the purpose of educating the patient.

Since it is considered as education, it should not be restricted to limited patients. It should cover as many patients as possible so as to achieve the best clinical outcome of the treatment.

Time of Counseling

The counseling is usually done at the end of a long course of treatment right before discharge. However, that is not a hard and fast rule. The counseling can also be done at the beginning or in the middle of the treatment, depending upon the patient's requirements. During the patient medication history interview, all the necessary information about the patient is gathered whereas the information is given during counseling. After the diagnosis, the treating physician gives some outline about the disease suspected and the probable treatment and duration. In case the patient requires more, a counseling session is conducted. Similarly, during the treatment, in order to ascertain the patient's feelings about their disease, its severity, comfort, problems in medicine usage, etc, a counseling session is conducted.

At the end of the treatment, just before the discharge, the patient is instructed about the continuation of the treatment in their homes, dos and don'ts regarding diet, exercise, repeat visit to the hospital, etc. This session of counseling is worthwhile because, after discharge, the patient loses the supervision of a doctor, pharmacist, or nurse. This often results in a careless attitude leading to a relapse of the disease or more complications.

The patients usually don't share all the details with their doctors regarding their medication habits. By counseling, a good counselor can get them to talk about what they'd usually hide by winning their confidence. Thus, counseling is beneficial to both the health care team and the patients.

Need for Counseling and Privacy

Counseling involves a two-way exchange of information between the pharmacist and the patient. Needless to mention, it is better than written communication. Moreover, legally and morally, pharmacists have to give information about the drugs that the patients use. It should cover all the necessary details and in the language that patients understand. Hence, counseling is inevitable. For effective counseling, the place must be free from noise, interruption or any possible distractions. Offering such privacy will help the patient understand its importance and gain cooperation. It also improves the image of the pharmacists and they will be recognized as the ones contributing to the patient welfare. Generally, the disease is private to the patient and they are naturally hesitant to discuss it openly. With infallible privacy, they tend to speak more about their inner problems and feelings.

Classification

Counseling can be classified into two types:

1. Direct counseling (face to face) and

2. Distant counseling, through phone

Although direct counseling is the one advised, distant counseling can also be useful for patients who can not visit the hospitals or clinics owing to their disease, immobility, or other problems. In developed countries, such services are available with a small fee that the patients themselves can opt for themselves. Usually, outpatients with chronic illness and elderly patients seek these services.

Suitable Person to Give Counseling

Generally, doctors, nurses, and pharmacists can conduct counseling for patients. However, the first two do not have the required time or environment for offering such services. As both doctors and nurses need to attend emergency cases at any time, their services remain confined to the ward. Moreover, waiting period, restlessness, anticipation, apprehension makes the patient reluctant to cooperate with counseling doctors. When in it comes to counseling by the nurses, the entire hospital setup including fellow patients and their disease complications, administration of different medications through a different route to other patients, various surgical instruments and apparatus present can affect the mindset of the patients regarding counseling. In these circumstances, the pharmacists are more suitable as they are away from this environment and are mostly available at all times. By the very nature of their jobs, they are experts in human relations (HR) and have knowledge about drugs and their side effects. Thus, pharmacists can take care of patients' needs and direct them suitably.

Special cases that require counseling

Routine counseling of all patients is both impossible and unnecessary. The patients are selected according to their needs. For some, a few minutes of counseling is sufficient and given during regular ward rounds or at the time of administration of drugs. But relatively longer counseling sessions are needed for the following people:

A. Patients to be subjected to long term treatment e.g.: Epilepsy cases.

B. Patients with diseases but without severe symptoms e.g.: Prophylactic cases of TB.

C. Patients using drugs with a narrow therapeutic index. e.g.: Warfarin.

D. Patients with the danger of abrupt stopping of treatment. e.g.: Corticosteroid therapy and

E. Patients with potential for non-compliance, abuse or misuse of drugs. e.g.: Treatment with tranquilizers.

Steps involved in counseling or preparation for counseling

Patient education and counseling can be carried out in all types of pharmacy practice, viz, inpatient care, outpatient care, home care and community care settings. However, counseling requires some prior preparation to be useful to the patient and to the institution.

Preparation for Counseling

It differs among the four settings mentioned above. If the counseling is for an inpatient at the time of discharge, the required information about the patient can be obtained from hospital records. However, if the counseling is to be carried out at the time admission of the patient, few days after the admission, for an outpatient, or in community pharmacy settings, the pharmacist should gather all the relevant information about the patient before starting counseling. If a pharmacist could acquire knowledge about the patient's cultures, especially their health and illness beliefs, attitude and practices, it goes a long way in dealing with them. If the counseling is done after a few days of admission and in the middle of the treatment, the counseling has to be in a different plain altogether. This is done to ensure that the patients realize their diseases can be cured if they adhere to the instructions of the health care team. In this scenario, getting their co-operation may not be a problem. In the hope to get better sooner, they tend to overlook issues like frequent injections, lab procedures, too many bitter tablets, etc. Similarly, effective counseling can help outpatients realize that these instructions are for their well-being only. Hence, for the counseling to be successful, the pharmacist should prepare themselves for all the repercussions involved.

As there is no effective supervision of the patient after discharge, proper counseling is required to prevent relapse and readmission of the patient. The appropriate learning aids like graphics, anatomical models, medication devices, memory aids, printed pamphlets, and audiovisual resources should always be available in the counseling room.

All this apart, while getting ready for counseling, the pharmacist should review the discharge prescription, ensure a clear medication list and all the instructions for discharge. The patient follow-up plan should also be handy. As mentioned above, a fairly good idea about the patient to be counseled can be collected from hospital records. The patient may be a child, elderly, mentally or terminally ill. Depending on the type of patient, the pharmacist should plan the counseling content. For example, a prior idea about their level of understanding is important to counsel children. On the other hand, an elderly patient may be vision or hearing impaired, a terminally ill patient may not be interested in counseling at all and may not pay attention during the session while a mentally ill patient may not understand and co-operate during the counseling. Before counseling, a pharmacist must be prepared to face all the possible situations.

Scope of counseling or contents of counseling

The scope or purpose of patient counseling is for providing instructions, motivation to patients and monitoring them in the process. The counseling for outpatients differs from the counseling for inpatients. To inpatients, certain points like how to open or administer drugs, timing and amount of dose, etc need not be discussed as they are taken care of by nurses. Those instructions should only be given at the time of discharge along with storage conditions, refill information, etc. However, all this information has to be conveyed to outpatients, detailing possible side effects, what to do in case of missing dosage, and the duration of treatment. For a complicated regimen like multiple drug regimen, complex packings, drugs have to be shown to the patient and explained.

This, not only makes them understand better but also helps the pharmacist in the detection of dispensing or prescription error. A few words about the use and importance of each drug will lead to better compliance and consequent success of the treatment.

Moreover, patients might be interested in knowing the expected duration of the treatment and the expected benefits. All this can be briefly mentioned while discussing the importance of adhering to the instructions. Furthermore, a possible drug-drug interaction and drug-food interaction should also be informed beforehand. The technique of self-monitoring of treatment should be taught to the patient. Depending on the patient's disease management and therapeutic plan, it is important to educate the patient regarding the disease state, its effects on normal life, and the identification of disease manifestations.

Before ending the counseling session, patients may be encouraged to speak their minds regarding the treatment. This is very important because there are many unanswered questions, misunderstandings, and problems that they may not reveal to the health care team. In the absence of answers to these problems, they make their own decisions regarding the treatment. When prompted, they tend to open up and ask questions and share their experiences with the treatment.

After clearing the patient's doubts, the pharmacist can ask a few questions at the end to estimate the patient's level of understanding and knowledge about counseling points. If required, the pharmacist can once again clarify their doubts with materials and demonstrations.

At any point in time, the pharmacist should not assume that the patient has understood all the information given and they will contact on their own in case of a problem. Also, they should not rely on the possibility of someone else from the health care team giving out the information to the patients in the ward.

Effects or Uses of Counseling

With the help of counseling:

1. Knowledge of disease and its treatment among the patients is improved.
2. Patient compliance is improved.
3. Repetition of drugs in use can be avoided.
4. Pharmacists' contribution to disease documentation is increased.
5. Since compliance is improved, the disease aggravation is reduced and
6. Because of it, an emergency visit to the hospital or hospitalization or subsequent expenses is also greatly reduced.

Thus, counseling plays an important role in disease management. Hence, for counseling clinical pharmacists should be appointed in all Indian hospitals.

Barriers or Problems in Patient Counseling

Though there are many advantages to patient counseling, in practice, it has several barriers. Following are some of the problems associated with it:

1. **Hospital Environment:** The hospital ward environment is not always suitable for patient counseling. Unless the patient is admitted to a separate room called a special ward, it is not conducive to go for counseling in a crowded general ward where dozens of other patients are admitted in beds close to each other. There is no privacy and hence, the patient may not openly discuss their problems, doubts, and observations of their body conditions. Also, the noise or sound level in the general ward is distracting and it is especially difficult for the patient to raise their voice. The remedy is to take the patient, even in a wheelchair, to a separate counseling room in the hospital. If it is not available, there must be at least one common room for two wards that can be used for counseling.

2. **Language Barrier:** A lot of patients in the govt. hospitals come from poor families and they are the ones that actually require counseling. But the majority of them only know their mother tongue and the use of English and technical terms during counseling can make it useless. Hence, the counseling pharmacist should able to speak in the language that the patient understands.

3. **Educational Level:** It is the fallout of the above situation where the patient's education level is poor. Hence, they may not be in a position to read the label or written instructions given to them. Even if they can read it, comprehending that information can be difficult for these patients.

4. **Disabilities of the body:** Many patients are in their advanced age and their eyesight and hearing abilities are below normal. Such patients have to be counseled with written materials

if they are able to read or with sign language if they can see it. The instructions must be repeated during counseling until the patient understands them.

5. **Patient motivation:** It is one of the important factors. Unless the patient is motivated and willing enough to cooperate, any amount of counseling can go to waste. The lack of motivation can be owed to multiple factors like a chronic illness, pending treatment, or depression. Some patients at the tail end of their life tend to show disinterest in counseling. The clinical pharmacists should understand it and conduct counseling sessions based on ground realities.

6. **Inadequate time or training:** Usually senior, experienced clinical pharmacists are assigned the duty of patient counseling. But on some rare occasions or at the time of training, juniors may be allotted the task of counseling the patients. This may reflect on the quality of counseling. Sometimes, due to lack of time or other pressing engagements, the clinical pharmacists tend to cut short the counseling sessions and that is also considered as one of the major barriers in counseling.

QUESTIONS

1. Write briefly about the need for Patient Counseling

2. What makes a pharmacist suitable to give Counseling?

3. What is the scope for Counseling?

4. List the uses of Counseling

5. List all the types patients that need counseling

6. Write a note on the barriers of Counseling.

7. How will you counsel a patient?

8. Write an essay about Patient Counseling

9. Conduct a mock Counseling using one of your classmates as a patient, document it, and submit.

CHAPTER **14**

EDUCATION AND TRAINING PROGRAM IN THE HOSPITAL

LEARNING OBJECTIVE

The objective of the chapter is to provide an overall picture of the education and training program in the hospital. However, it includes other related aspects like interdepartmental communication and code of ethics for community pharmacy as per the syllabus. Hence a reader can have a bird's eye view about the topic

ROLE OF HOSPITAL PHARMACIST IN EDUCATION AND TRAINING

INTRODUCTION

As the graduate and post-graduate pharmacists are educated and trained in dealing with almost all drug-related aspects, they are experts in the field of their specialization drugs. They not only study the pharmacological properties of drugs but also about their physical, chemical, and pharmaceutical properties. It is safe to conclude that their knowledge about drugs is out-and-out which makes them well qualified to teach about drugs. They can teach student nurses, pharmacists, medical students, and house surgeons about the practical aspects of drug usage. The pharmacists can also educate social workers, patients and also people in general.

Internal Teaching Program

When the pharmacists teach the hospital staff and students, it is referred to as an internal teaching program. For instance, by the nature of their jobs, the nurses are not given extensive coverage of pharmacology during their course of study. Hence, any addition to that knowledge can be appreciated. The study material is prepared by the teaching pharmacists to explain specific topics that can be taught and discussed in classes, specially arranged for them.

Similarly, seminars can be arranged for medical staff and graduate nurses on topics like hospital formulary, prescription errors, incompatibilities in IV admixture, new drug regulations, drug-drug interactions, and more. In addition to printed literature, brochures, including slide shows, short films, and other audiovisual materials in the session can make the teaching method more effective. These materials can be procured from WHO, pharmaceutical manufacturers, or simply be prepared using the internet at the drug information center attached to the hospital.

In order to disseminate hands-on practical knowledge, new drugs and updated packings of old drugs can also be shown to the participants. The continuing education programs for working pharmacists and health care teams are an ideal example of teaching for staff.

Teaching Patients and/or their Attendants

It may not be possible to teach patients while they are sick and still undergoing treatment, however, they can be educated at the time of discharge. The majority of patients are given medicines along with a set of instructions at the time of discharge. Unless they are educated via counseling, the disease may relapse. Hence, a suitable program to educate the patients, as well as their caretakers, can go a long way in monitoring the post-discharge medications and symptoms. The instructions of general nature, such as, how to identify adverse drug effects can be given to a group of patients via short lectures or closed-circuit television programs.

External Teaching Programs

The External Teaching Programs consist of teaching activities performed by the pharmacists outside their hospitals. Conducting seminars, participating as a resource person in refresher courses, delivering lectures in clubs and association meetings are all part of external teaching programs. For medical and paramedical professionals, seminars can be conducted over various topics like the latest drug profiles, new adverse drug reactions, and substitutes available for problem drugs, etc. These teaching programs are especially appreciated by the nursing, dietary and lab technology people as they add so much to their knowledge.

Similarly, senior pharmacists can work on the real external teaching program of educating and refreshing the knowledge of working pharmacists. Periodically, these refresher programs are conducted by pharmacy colleges in collaboration with State Pharmacy Councils. These programs could include various topics related to the latest developments in the pharmacy field that can be of interest to the working pharmacists who may not have the time to read professional journals due to their pressing workload and lack of resources.

In addition to this, senior pharmacists, especially those who are professors in teaching hospitals are always in demand at the elite clubs like the Lions Club and the Rotary clubs. They invite teaching professionals to contribute to their association's regular monthly meetings. In some cities, there are few other elite associations for senior and retired government officers of various departments who have the time and capability to understand technical and scientific matters about drugs. Since the majority of them are using one or the other drug due to their age-related issues, they are very eager and receptive to the lectures by senior pharmacists. The author of this book had few such opportunities and enjoyed post-lecture interactions with the said audience, and thereby, have first-hand information regarding the whereabouts of such lectures.

Furthermore, the pharmacists can also teach in writing in addition to conducting full-blown seminars. They can prepare manuscripts for publication in professional journals. They can also contribute via educational pamphlets, posters or display materials to educate the patients as well as the general public. Thus, there are immense opportunities for a pharmacist to involve in an external teaching program.

Community Health Education

The pharmacists can indulge in outside lecture assignments on general or specific topics and educate the people in general. They can participate in seminars and lectures arranged by social service organizations like Lions Club, Rotary Club, etc. Pamphlets and posters can go a long way in educating the general public in large numbers at a time. If possible, the pharmacists should organize such programs for rural masses where the poor and illiterate people need to be educated to eradicate superstitions about diseases and bad treatment practices. An audio-visual method of communication is more suitable for rural people. This could include cinema, drama and other art forms like street corner short plays to serve the purpose. The pharmacists can write scripts for these methods of education. Drug abuse prevention is one major teaching program where pharmacists can contribute a lot with their knowledge and experience. Above all, the pharmacists can write general articles on topics like dangers of antibiotic resistance, misuse or abuse of drugs, self medications, etc in professional and news journals, and magazines.

Training

A suitable training program must be drawn for student pharmacists, by the hospital and community pharmacists. Apart from the usual dispensing practices, the students should be trained in all aspects of stores and dispensary management. Starting from the drug purchase procedure to storage, distribution, and accounting, they should be trained under the chief or senior pharmacists. At the end of the training, they should be evaluated for adequate knowledge and then certified for the same. Similarly, student nurses and doctors can also be trained in specific aspects of proper methods of use, storage, and disposal of dangerous and other important drugs.

Services to Nursing Homes and Clinics

The concept of outside pharmacists providing services to nursing homes and clinics is new and not practiced in India. However, knowing that such services exist in other countries helps the pharmacists to either adopt them or when they choose to go abroad.

In India, pharmacists are not appointed in small clinics and nursing homes. Their tasks are carried out by non-pharmacists, especially nurses and other trained people. In our country, the doctors have the legal authority to dispense medicines to their patients. So, the question of appointing pharmacists or engaging the services of outside pharmacists does not arise. As long as this is in practice, the professional services by pharmacists in nursing homes and clinics will remain non-existent.

Only recently, the govt. of India has brought an Act called 'Clinical establishments Act', according to which, the nursing homes and hospitals should maintain certain standards in regards to facilities, staff, and infrastructure to get registration under the act. The full implementation of this act is still awaited as many of the state governments have neither adopted this central act nor implemented an act of their own. So, we can't do anything but wait for full or part-time pharmacy services in clinics and nursing homes. In the meantime, let us learn more about such services available abroad.

In the USA, the term 'Nursing Home' is defined as a facility or a unit that is designated, staffed, and equipped for the accommodation of individuals who do not require hospital care but nursing and other medical services. These are performed under the direction of professionals that are licensed to provide such care and services in accordance with the laws of the state in which the facilities are located.

In these nursing homes and clinics, the pharmacists are appointed either on a part-time basis or on a contract basis. In either case, the following facilities are provided in the nursing homes:

1. A compact, adequate, separate drug room

2. A pharmacist on active duty in the hospital on an average of 3 hours per day

3. Telephone service, to be used for consultation and order placement with an outside pharmacy and

4. A standby delivery service from outside [community] pharmacy to the nursing home.

Functions of part-time pharmacists in nursing homes:

1. To furnish drugs of standard quality without supply interruptions

2. To maintain a record for the services provided to the patients

3. To procure and purchase drugs required for the nursing home and

4. To ensure safe medication practices in nursing homes by maintaining the patient's drug profile.

In India, small clinics that are established and run by a single doctor or a couple of additional doctors have fixed working hours. Their services are directed towards outpatient only. Here, the doctor writes the prescription and sends the patient to purchase the drugs from the nearby community pharmacies. So, that eliminates the need for pharmacists in these clinics.

On the other hand, if provision for admitting the patients in a few beds in these nursing homes and small hospitals is established, they have round the clock nursing services and other supportive services. Here, a pharmacy may be established by appointing part-time or full-time pharmacists.

Thus, a pharmacist can serve the nursing homes as a full time or a part-time employee, depending on requirements. It is important to note that irrespective of the position, the pharmacists have to perform all the usual professional services expected from him.

Code of Ethics for Community Pharmacy

A community pharmacy is not just an organization of service but also a business entity. They sell medicines and other health care needs for a price with some margin of profit, which is essential for their survival. However, the medicine business is different from the businesses of other commodities. It needs to follow some ethics in its dealings with patients and the public. Such ethics are framed by the Pharmacy Council of India and the pharmacists are strictly advised to follow them. They are discussed below:

1. **Price structure:** Though the prices of all drugs are printed on the label, community pharmacy needs to follow them in letter and spirit. The maximum retail price inclusive of all taxes is printed on all the labels and containers of the medicine but they are not followed when the packing is opened and fractions of its content are sold in loose to the customers. Some pharmacies with legal permission also collect service charges from the customers. However, those service charges should be reasonable and proportionate to the service offered.

2. **Far trade practice:** On any account, the community pharmacies should not indulge in cut-throat competition with neighboring pharmacies. They should not follow any deep-discount strategies or schemes to attract customers and maintain the business. Similarly, they should not imitate the labels, trademarks, symbols, logos of the contemporary pharmacies. If the prescription for a particular pharmacy is brought to it by mistake, they should immediately direct it to the correct pharmacy.

3. **Purchase of drugs:** Drugs and other medical devices should always be purchased from genuine and authorized suppliers. Under no circumstances, unauthorized sources should be encouraged by placing orders. There is a great possibility that the medicines offered at very low prices come from illegal sources with questionable content and substandard. Even if genuine original drugs are offered with a heavy discount without an invoice, the source must be questioned. They might have been smuggled or stolen from the original manufacturer. Hence, a community pharmacist must be vigilant and information regarding any malpractice should be forwarded to drugs control department or police.

4. **Hawking of drugs:** Under any circumstances, a community pharmacy should not involve hawking of drugs. It is a bad practice to solicit orders by canvassing the neighborhood door to door. It not only lowers the status of the pharmacists but also leads to misuse or abuse of drugs which subsequently spoils the society at large.

5. **Advertising and displays:** It is natural for any business to advertise their commodities and services. But for medicines, this practice must be within the ethical parameters. The advertisements should not reflect unfavorably on competitive pharmacies, clinics or fellow individuals. It should not also favour them. Misleading or exaggerated statements or claims should be avoided. There should be no claim for the efficacy of the medicines sold or refund in the case of failure. The content of the advertisement should be decent. It should not refer to sexual weakness, impotency, premature aging, etc.

Thus the community pharmacy must convey a professional image to the community at large and to its customers in particular by following the ethics.

Role of Pharmacist in Interdepartmental Communication

During the course of the practice of their profession, pharmacists have to communicate with several people like the prescribers, patients and their helpers, nurses, drug suppliers, colleagues, and higher officials. On a few occasions, they adopt written communication with these people, especially with higher officials and other departments of the same hospital or outside. If they initiate communication with colleagues in other departments of the same institution, it is referred to as interdepartmental communication.

This communication may be for many reasons on multiple subjects. For example, the majority of these communications are an invitation to the seminar, conferences, and other society-related activities of the pharmacy department. Other communications are for requesting services and materials from these departments. Few others are for passing on information about new drugs, new dosage forms old drugs, ADR, etc. via newsletters and bulletin.

Irrespective of the content of the communication, the style, language, and format should be polite and dignified. They can look up the format for "How to write an official letter" to help them with the same. Similarly, letters received from other departments should be properly numbered, filed, and replied to in an appropriate manner. Drafting a good letter is something that a pharmacist must learn at any cost. These well-written letters bring in a prompt and positive response from the department concerned, thereby, helping the pharmacists in the smooth running of the pharmacy and the department.

Interdepartmental communications may happen frequently in a dispensary or a hospital but there are substantial communications among the medical and surgical stores sections, purchase section and Chief Pharmacist's desk. Hence, student [trainee] pharmacists should be smart enough to learn the technique of Interdepartmental communications from senior pharmacists.

QUESTIONS

1. Write a note on community health education

2. Enumerate the internal teaching program of a hospital pharmacist

3. Write briefly about the pharmacist's services to nursing homes and clinics

4. What are the ethics that should be followed by Community Pharmacists?

5. Write about Interdepartmental communication in detail.

CHAPTER 15

PRESCRIBED MEDICATION ORDER AND COMMUNICATION SKILLS

LEARNING OBJECTIVE

Learn the difference between prescription and prescribed medication order, Know the types of medication order, Understand how communication skill is important in pharmacy and How to communicate with patients

The prescribed medication order is nothing but a prescription written by a registered medical practitioner. However, there is a difference between prescription and medication order. Prescriptions are given to the outpatients whereas medication orders are for the inpatients. The prescription medication order doesn't require in-depth instructions as the mentioned drugs are to be administered in a ward setting by nurses and pharmacists. On the other hand, prescriptions require full detail instructions to the patient as they are going to take those medicines without any supervision by a health care professional.

However, these differences are not recognized by many health care professionals including pharmacists and they often use these terms interchangeably which results in confusion. Let us dive into details of both the concepts. Logically thinking, the name prescription medication order has the word 'order' in it, which is generally issued by superiors to their subordinates in an institutional setting. An order cannot be issued to an outsider [like community pharmacist] and the word has an inherent hegemony which is not appreciated. Hence, a prescription is the apt word for the requirement of drugs for an outpatient.

Prescribed Medication Order as Inpatient Prescription

A medication order is otherwise known as a drug order or a physician's order. These orders have similar instructions as in the prescription except for a few differences. They have the patient's hospital ID number, date of admission, and provision for the pharmacist's and the nurse's note which is missing in prescriptions.

Different hospitals follow a different procedure to get the medicines for the inpatients. In our country, these medication orders are written on the punch of case sheets hanging on the patient's bed during the ward rounds by the treating physician. They are then noted on the prescription sheets by ward nurse and after getting the initials from the physician concerned, they are taken to the ward pharmacy or the main medical store of the hospital for dispensing by pharmacists. The nurses receive the medicine on behalf of inpatients and administer as per the dose and time mentioned in the medication order. This method of dispensing is followed in almost all govt. hospitals. Alternatively, the nurses give the prescription to the patient's attender and ask them to collect medicines from the pharmacy attached to the hospital. It is kept in the bedside table of the patient for administration as when due. This method is followed in private hospitals.

PRESCRIBED MEDICATION ORDER SHEET

HOSPITAL NAME AND ADDRESS

PATIENT NAME: AGE/SEX

HOSPITAL.ID No.

DATE OF ADMISSION:

WARD: BED No.

DIAGNOSIS:

ALLERGY: NURSE'S NOTE

DATE   TIME   HOUR   INITIAL

1   [DRUGS NAME, DOSE & INSTRUCTION]

2

3

DOCTOR'S SIGNATURE:

Types of medication orders

There are four types of medication orders: 1. Stat 2.Single 3.Standing and 4. PRN orders.

1. The stat order is issued in emergency cases. It means the drug should be administered as soon as possible but only once. For example Diazepam 10 mg IV stat for patients with seizures.

2. The single order is the for one-time administration of the drug. Example: Furosemide 20 mg IV to be given one time at 7 am

3. The standing order is for a medicine to be given for a specified number of doses. For example, Cefazolin 1g q 6H x doses until discontinued. However, many hospitals have

policies to stop all the drugs after a specific number of doses unless a renewal order is written and

4. A PRN order is one for the drug to be administered if needed.

Prescribed Medication Order as an Outpatient Prescription

Outpatient prescriptions are not only issued in private practice by Registered Medical Practitioners but also to the patients visiting government hospitals for their short term problems which do not require hospitalization. Irrespective of the origin of the prescription, it needs to be dispensed correctly. WHO has recommended some steps in its guidance under the topic 'Good Dispensing Practice' [GDP] which is quoted below:

There are 4 steps in dispensing prescribed drugs.

1. Screening 2. Interpretation 3. Getting clarification and 4.Dispensing extra-ordinary prescriptions.

As per the government, the Medical Council of India and its guidance document 'Medical Manual', there should be stipulated minimum detail about the patients and the drugs prescribed in all prescriptions. A pharmacist must first screen the prescription for the above details as they are the legal requirements.

Step 1. Screening: A] Check: Is the prescription issued for the correct patient and according to the act and rules? B] Is it written legibly or printed? C] It has no abbreviations used D] Weather the age and body weight of the children below 12 years is mentioned?

Step 2. Interpretation: Check for A] Dose, its frequency and duration. If excess or double dose is written deliberately and whether it is underlined?   B] Possible drug interaction, Medicine duplication, inappropriate drug therapy, and contra indications.C] Allergy D] unusual usage, suspected misuse or abuse. The pharmacist should also check for the maximum dose and duration of a particular drug if it is supplied in installments as per the prescription.

Step 3. Clarification: If any clarification is needed in the prescription, the prescriber should be contacted. If they are available, the pharmacist should arrange for inserting missing detail by the prescriber and should discuss remedial action. If the prescriber is not available in the hospital, the pharmacist should get the authorization to make corrections over the phone. They should write *"Prescriber contacted over the phone"* on the back of the prescription and put their initials and date. If the pharmacist is not able to contact the prescriber, they should send back the prescription asking for clarification. Similarly, approval of the prescriber is needed for substitution of the drug and the same should be documented on the prescription.

Step 4. Extraordinary Prescription: These are the prescriptions for poisons and psychotropic drugs. There are some legal requirements for dispensing these prescriptions that should be strictly followed.

A] For poison: The issue of poison should be recorded in a separate book for poisons on the day of supply itself. The book for poison should have the following particulars: date of supply, the serial number of entry, name of the medicine and its quantity, name, and address of the patient and name and address of the prescriber with register number.

B] For Psychotropic Drugs: the separate book for these drugs should contain all the above information. In addition, it should have a separate page for each psychotropic drug where quantity issued and balance on hand should be recorded immediately after the sale. All these records should be in the form of a bound book. If computer printouts are taken, they should be made into a bound book.

COMMUNICATION SKILLS

Why it is important?

According to F.Rabinson, " communicating, and doing it well is vital to building relationships with your patients, delivering successful interventions, consultations, and improving health outcomes". Poor communication with patients leads to non-compliance with the instructions and results in a greater risk of complications. Hence, the pharmacist must communicate directly with the patient or the prescriber to ensure that the prescribed therapy is fully understood. It should never be assumed that the patient knows the proper use.

Communication barriers

There are some barriers to good communication. A pharmacist must overcome such barriers to be a successful practitioner. One major barrier is the lack of training. A pharmacist should consult with other healthcare professionals to get different views on patient care. The lack of such interprofessional training leads to the failure in providing useful pharmaceutical care to the patients. Other barriers are multiple prescribers and their unavailability for consultation. The patients go to different practitioners for their different problems which may be concurrent. They end up taking multiple drugs at a time, sometimes even from the alternative systems of medicine. Hence, there is a higher possibility of drug-drug interaction. To foresee such interaction, a pharmacist should communicate well with patients and the other prescribers, if possible. The pharmacist's workload also acts as a barrier to communication.

How to improve communication skills?

Basic subject knowledge is essential for effective communication. If you are ignorant of a subject, you tend to speak less. A pharmacist must be a continuous learner. They should gather knowledge from professional journals, books, and literature supplied by medical representatives. They can find time for reading by avoiding and delegating non-professional tasks to the assistants.

The shortest way to learn is to listen to the professional lectures and noting down the key points. Most of the information is available on the internet. An inclination towards learning from the digital sources will save time and trouble. The next method of improving a skill is by practice and experience. In their professional activities, pharmacists have to deal with patients, prescribers, medical representatives and other health care professionals. Communication with these people definitely improves the communication skill of the pharmacist and the same is discussed in detail below:

Communication with patients:

1] During Drug Administration or Dispensing:

While giving drugs to the patients, pharmacists must communicate effectively with them. Their voices must be clear, louder and understandable. Pharmacists should be able to make the patient understand the instructions. Improper and half-hearted communication results in grave error. Also, it is more important to communicate effectively in a simple language in our country where a large number of people with low literacy levels are using government hospitals and community pharmacies for their treatment. Depending on the patient's condition, age, and literacy level, we may have to follow a written communication system as well. Sometimes, the diagrams of tablets and capsules may have to be drawn to indicate the number of doses per day. This helps in reducing errors by the patients.

A pharmacist must be thorough with the common terms (medical and non-medical) used in the clinical practice of the hospital. They should also understand the abbreviations used by medical staff in prescriptions and other records so as to communicate effectively with colleagues and patients.

Sometimes, pharmacists do not communicate enough with the patients owing to various reasons like workload, fatigue, surrounding noise, and other disturbances. However, it is a law in the USA and other developed countries that pharmacists must communicate with patients to review the drug use and offer to counsel. They must discuss the following with each patient:

1. Name and description of medicine they dispense.
2. Dosage form, dose, routes of administration, and the duration of the drug therapy.
3. Special directions and precautions for preparation, administration, and use by the patient.
4. Side effects, adverse effects, interaction and contraindications of the drug and the ways of avoiding them, action required if they occur.
5. The technique of self-monitoring of drug therapy.
6. Proper storage
7. Prescription refill information
8. Action to be taken if a dose or two is missed
9. Instruction regarding the use of medical/surgical appliances and
10. Disposal of unused medicines, if any.

2] During Medication History Interview

A clinical pharmacist has to obtain an accurate medication history from the patient. This is not an easy task due to various reasons like the patient's physical and mental conditions. They can be sick, nervous, excited and also the questions asked during this interview are mostly personal in nature. Hence, they are reluctant to disclose everything honestly. So, it requires great communication abilities on the part of the clinical pharmacists to put clever questions without offending the patient's feelings. Once, they are able to convince the patient about the intention and usefulness of the information in diagnosis and treatment, a healthy relationship is built between them, resulting in a successful interview.

3] During Monitoring of Therapy

The primary duty of a clinical pharmacist is the monitoring of drug therapy. To do this effectively, the patient's understanding of instructions must be checked. Only the correct understanding leads to proper compliance with the instructions. Hence, by communicating with the patient, the pharmacist has to verify it. This leads to the identification of patient's practices during the course of treatment which leaves the room for making corrections in those practices. By close interaction with the patient, the pharmacist can identify any side effects, ADR, and drug interactions. All these works, points to the need for good communication skills.

4] During Patient Counseling

While counseling someone, you need to have empathy, consideration, and above all, good communication skills in order to make the patient follow your advice. The patients are counseled either during treatment or after discharge and sometimes on both occasions. The former counseling leads to the identification of factors that reduce compliance and the latter leads to the prevention of any chance of non- compliance after discharge. During counseling, the pharmacist must identify and deal with information deficiency, patient emotions, and functional limitations to ensure that the patients understand and carry out the instructions properly. All these require better communication and its importance is evident.

Communication with prescribers

During the course of their practice of the profession, pharmacists have to often communicate with the prescriber regarding various aspects of prescription, diagnosis, stock, storage, purchase, disposal and dispensing of drugs. In the community pharmacy practice, this communication is limited to the above aspects. However, in the hospital pharmacy practice, a pharmacist has to discuss a lot of other matters as well. These include the purchase of new drugs, pharmacy budget, the requirement for special camps, etc. However, such matters arise once in a while. The day to day communication mainly revolves around the patient's prescriptions and clarification on them.

As mentioned earlier, a pharmacist should get clarification from the prescriber in case of any doubts. Under any circumstances, they should not guess and assume the prescriber's intent. If they are not able to contact them, they can make notations on the back of the prescription and send back the patient to the prescriber. Thus, if verbal communication is not possible at the moment, a form of written communication should be initiated.

Politely, they can point out any discrepancies in the prescription without offending the feelings of the prescriber or the patient. In fact, a busy prescriber welcomes such help from pharmacists as long as the communication is useful to all concerned. Hence, a pharmacist should not hesitate to initiate a dialogue with the prescribers.

The pharmacists can also start such communication on their own regarding the arrival of new drugs, new dosage forms, packing, price reduction, any adverse report about a drug and consequent non-availability of such drugs. They can also pass any relevant information from the drug control department to the doctor. Such timely information goes a long way in the perfection of prescriber's medical practice. Thus, mutual respect, cooperation, trust, and rapport develops between the prescriber and pharmacist.

QUESTIONS

1. What is the prescribed medication order?

2. What are the types of medication order?

3. What is communication?

4. What are communication skills?

5. How should you improve communication skills?

6. Explain the importance of communication in pharmacy.

7. What are the points a pharmacist has to communicate during dispensing? Add a note on communications with prescribers

8. What are the 4 steps in dispensing prescribed drugs?

Chapter **16**

BUDGET PREPARATION AND IMPLEMENTATION

LEARNING OBJECTIVE

On complete reading of the chapter, the student should able to explain all aspects of budget preparation, including its divisions, requirements, factors affecting it, etc. By using that knowledge he should able to assist the budget preparation of his office wherever he gets employment or prepare it himself if self-employed.

INTRODUCTION

A new pharmacist, on joining duty in a hospital pharmacy, is not required to prepare the annual budget of the department. However, they are expected to learn about their department's important tasks that majorly involves budget preparation and its implementation. It determines the overall performance of the hospital pharmacy for the next year and beyond.

The budget of the hospital pharmacy is one of the most important things to consider. Hence, any deficiency in its preparation and implementation will reflect on the reputation of the entire hospital. Thus, it becomes all the more important that a realistic budget is prepared by taking into consideration all factors, circumstances, and the success of the previous budget or otherwise.

DEFINITION

A budget is nothing but a plan for future operations in financial terms. The plan is prepared, according to the financial implication of all functions of the hospital pharmacy. Thus, the budget is an instrument to review the working of any department by higher authorities in relation to the prepared plan, in a comprehensive and integrated manner that is expressed in financial terms.

As the overall hospital budget is the combination of all its departmental budgets, it must be prepared with the utmost sincerity. So, a pharmacist must be aware of what their department aims to achieve and then its divisions and the factors that would affect the budget.

Aim or Objectives of Budget

1. It sets a goal to be achieved and the standards for the department's performance.

2. By comparing the actual results with the goal in the midway appraisal of the budget helps to identify failures.

3. By analyzing the failures, the mistakes can be corrected beforehand

If a budget is not prepared, the above objectives cannot be achieved resulting in the shutdown of the organizations.

Factors Affecting Budget

A budget has to be prepared primarily according to the needs of a department but it is not as simple as it appears to be. The budget is influenced by multiple factors like local conditions and compulsions, management's policies and pressures, higher authorities' confidence in the department's ability and the head of the department's skill in the implementation of the budget.

1. **Local conditions and compulsions:** A budget prepared without taking local needs into consideration will be problematic during implementation. The local community is the beneficiary of the budget, and hence, their needs should be given priority while preparing a budget. For example, in a place where water-borne diseases are more, the drugs for those diseases should be purchased in needed quantity and budget provisions should be made for its purchase. Otherwise, there will be interim local purchases, making the annual budget useless. In order to prepare a useful budget, the knowledge of demographic, epidemiological, and attitudinal characters of the local community is essential. This is why the local people's representatives like MLA or MC are included in the consultative or advisory committee of the hospital.

2. **Management's policy:** The budget has to be prepared in accordance with the policies and the objectives of the management. These policies are not always constant and sometimes change out of pressure. Accordingly, the budget and programs of pharmacy services should be prepared. They should coincide with the overall plan of the institution. For example, the management may change its policy towards pricing the drugs. Hence, the drugs suitable for charging have to be procured. Similarly, for handing out free of charge, drugs at optimum prices should be purchased from the manufacturer. All these factors change the budget that was prepared earlier. Overall, the budget allocation for drug purchases has to be either increased or decreased according to the new policies.

3. **Confidence of higher authorities:** Being out and out money-related, the budget requires the confidence of higher authorities and trust on the budget preparing and implementing department. The previous year's performance is taken into account while according sanction to the current year's budget. As the budget of the hospital pharmacy department is connected with supply and services to the other departments, the support from those department heads will also be useful in getting sanction for proposals of the pharmacy department.

4. **The ability of the head of pharmacy services**: In sanctioning the budget proposal, the ability and integrity of the head of the department of pharmacy are also considered. The personal reputation goes a long way towards achieving the goals of the department. As mentioned earlier, the successful completion and achievement of the target of the previous year's budget are the deciding factors for getting sanction for the proposed budget without cuts.

Requirement/Characters of a Budget

1. First of all, the management must define the policies and objectives of the budget, taking into consideration, the growth of the hospital.
2. These policies and objectives must be clearly understood by those in a managerial position, because without their active support and participation, the goals cannot be achieved.
3. The aims of the budget should be reasonable and achievable.
4. The departments' capability should not be misinterpreted and unachievable goals should not be focused. The prevailing and anticipated conditions should be estimated correctly.
5. The budget should not restrict staff initiatives or discourage them from attempting new ventures and practices.

Divisions of a Budget

A budget has many sections depending upon the money that comes in or out. Thus, it can be classified into (a) Revenue (income) accounts (b) Expense accounts, and (c) Capital accounts. The last two are dealing with money that goes out but with a little difference, the former involves expenses of recurring nature and the latter deals with one-time expenses and investment in assets.

(a) **Revenue accounts:** The revenue or income for the hospital pharmacy department comes through the sale of drugs to inpatients, outpatients, and other departments. While preparing the budget, the previous year's revenue has to be considered and the revenue for the forthcoming year has to be estimated. When calculating all this, risk factors like price rise, fall in demand, etc should be borne in mind. Another source of income for the department is from the sale of empty containers, bottles, and other packing materials which are generated in huge volumes in big hospitals. This apart, any professional service rendered to outside agencies by the departments can be levied a service charge and credited in the revenue account. The revenue generated by the pharmacy department of a charity or government hospital is minimum but it is a considerable amount in the private hospitals.

(b) **Expenses accounts:** It can be broadly classified into administrative expenses and professional expenses. The administrative expenses include salaries and wages, stationeries, telephone, and electricity bills for the office, etc. The professional expenses include drug purchase bills, raw materials and other supplies, expenses involved in the maintenance of professional equipment and instruments, etc. These expenses are known as recurring expenses as they are made repeatedly in a financial year and the forthcoming years.

The salaries and wages are calculated for all the employees of the department including the part-time and temporary employees. If new posts are to be created in the next financial year, the anticipated salary should also be added to this heading. Overtime wages, if any, to be paid to the employees should also be calculated. In these calculations, the previous year's experience in the working of the department offers valuable guidance.

Supply and expenses include all purchases to the department mainly the drugs and other pharmaceuticals and raw materials. Allowance should be made for future expansion, price rise and local and emergency purchases. While calculating the expected cost of purchase for the forthcoming year, taxes, transport expenses, insurance, loading and unloading charges, etc should not be forgotten.

(c) Capital accounts: Capital expenses are not recurring expenses and are considered as one-time expenses. The construction of new buildings, purchase of new equipments, etc fall under this category. Although these are assets added to the department, due to wear and tear, they depreciate in value in due course of time and have to be replaced. That might be a huge expense for the institute. Hence, depreciation value is detected from the revenue account and separately kept aside for future purchases. The depreciation value for each year is deducted, depending on the durability or life of the equipment or asset.

Deducting and setting aside depreciation value is irrelevant to the government hospitals, whereas it is a possibility in private hospitals. The head of the department of the pharmacy has to fix life periods of depreciable machinery and instruments in consultation with their manufacturers and suppliers. Only they can guarantee the serviceability in terms of years as this factor depends upon workmanship, quality control factors, and frequency or extent of usage of the equipment under question.

Usually, for small expenses, a unit cost of say Rs. 1000 may be fixed and any expense above this value is put under capital account after approval from the higher authorities. The sealing is deliberately kept low in order to have better control over the finances. The public health sector that includes the hospitals is considered 'white elephant' by higher officers of the finance ministry. In simple terms, it means, they incur only expenses and do not generate any income for the government. Hence, it is impossible for the hospitals to make any huge capital expense from its internal resources or the income generated by the hospital. Almost all the capital expenses are made by grants from the State or Central Government or the trust that manages the hospital.

Government Hospital Budgets (The Preparation Process)

The budget preparation processes are more or less the same for private hospitals and government hospitals. The budget prepared as above by the HOD of the hospital pharmacy should be submitted to the management in the case of private hospitals. Similarly, it is submitted to the higher authorities in the case of government hospitals. They, in turn, submit the consolidated budget of all sections of their organization to their higher authorities, well before the beginning of the budget session of parliament or state assembly in February every year. The budgets thus collected from all the hospitals of the district by District Medical Officer (DMO) or District Health Officer (DHO) are submitted to the state level directorates after corrections, if any and recommendations within their budget allocations. The State Director of Medical Services [DMS] or Health Services [DHS] or Medical Education [DME], in turn, consolidates all district-level budgets, include their own office's budget and then submit to the health ministry in the state secretariat. They forward these budget proposals with modifications, if any, to the finance ministry for final approval and also pass it in the state legislature during state budget for the forthcoming financial year.

Each and every budget proposal thus submitted is scrutinized by financial experts and senior officers at various levels, either approved in full or with cuts and sent back to the department concerned for implementation. This happens after the state assembly or parliament passes it before 31st March of every year.

Budget approval and implementation: From the above discussion, it is clear that the hospital pharmacy department is required to maintain somewhat detailed and correct records to arrive at the figures for the budget. Though it is very desirable to collect and keep one's own statistical data, in practice, it is commonly observed for the pharmacist to depend upon the accounts department for many basic figures.

Hence, the pharmacist must develop a close liaison with the accounts officer of the hospital so that they can prepare the best budget. Through its correct implementation, they earn a reputation for themselves and their department.

However, they should be ready to receive their budget proposals with cuts or modifications at the beginning of each financial year, say by April. They must implement it with full efficiency, so as to get the approval of the next budget proposals without any cuts.

QUESTIONS

1. List the objectives of Hospital Pharmacy Budget.

2. What are the characters of a budget?

3. How is a budget for the hospital pharmacy prepared?

4. Enumerate the factors affecting the budget of a hospital pharmacy.

5. What are the different sections of a budget? Explain.

CHAPTER 17

CLINICAL PHARMACY

LEARNING OBJECTIVE

This long chapter describes large number of aspects of clinical pharmacy practice, including its concept, basis, functions, drug therapy monitoring, medication chart review, individualization of dose, ward round participation, medication history interview, and pharmaceutical care. It also explains clinical review and pharmacist intervention, dosing pattern and drug therapy based on pharmacokinetic and disease patterns etc. A thorough reading and understanding of the chapter will initiate the student into clinical pharmacy practice.

INTRODUCTION

Clinical pharmacy is a new branch of pharmacy introduced in the health care system. It is well accepted and currently practiced in the USA, UK, Australia, and other developed countries where the pharmacists perform the clinical pharmacy services. Though this service was introduced in these countries decades back, it is yet to be started in India. With the increasing advancement in the field of science, it is a matter of time before it makes its way to India. Hence, today's pharmacy students have to be familiar with this subject.

Need / Concept of Clinical Pharmacy

What is the need for a clinical pharmacy? Why was suddenly a new branch of pharmacy started? How was the concept of clinical pharmacy evolved? All these questions need to be answered for the introduction of the subject.

In order to survive and make their way to the new markets, big pharmaceutical companies are spending millions of dollars in research and development of new drugs. As a result, new drugs are introduced into the market at regular intervals. Even before these drugs get acceptance and widespread use, another drug or formulation is introduced by the competing company, with claims of better actions. Thus, there are hundreds of potent new drugs, for the doctors to prescribe with the consequent risk of side effects, drug interactions, etc. The competition between the drug companies is such that they flood the market not only with new drugs but also with literature and information about those drugs with a lot of claims and counterclaims. Getting authentic and correct information from this junk is so difficult, and hence, an expert in drug information is needed.

Apart from this, we know that a doctor can allot very little time for each patient during the course of diagnosis and treatment. Also, many patients start using one or the other drug even before the treatment starts for the present or already existing diseases. This predisposes the patient for ill effects during either present or future therapy. Hence, the patient's medication history is essential before starting the treatment. A suitable specialist is needed for this job. This specialist should also be able to decide the appropriateness of the drug therapy, benefit to risk ratio, and alternative regimes if required.

We all have common anatomy but not common physiology i.e., the degree of functions of our internal organs differs from person to person. Hence, a generalized dose may not be suitable for all the patients. The patient's conditions differ widely from the complications they carry like diabetes, hypertension, kidney damage, liver damage, etc. Hence, an adjustment in the dose for each patient is required, which involves many calculations based on scientific studies on the patient and his body fluids. Thus, individualization of dose and selection of drugs to suit the particular individual has to be performed by an expert. If not, the treatment cannot be claimed as fully scientific, at best it can be semi-scientific or pseudo-scientific.

However, the immediate reason for the evolution of the concept of clinical pharmacy was the THALIDOMIDE disaster of 1960-1961. The drug, Thalidomide was developed in West Germany and marketed in several countries. It was given for controlling nausea and vomiting during the early stages of pregnancy and was available without the requirement of a prescription, as an OTC drug.

Thalidomide given to pregnant women produced 'PHOCOMELIA' – an arrested development of limbs of newborn infants. In West Germany alone, there were 10,000 birth deformities. The drug also affected thousands of infants in other countries such as England, Israel, Australia, Belgium, Brazil, Canada, East Germany, Egypt, Lebanon, Peru, Spain, Sweden, and Switzerland, totaling a few lakhs babies.

Thalidomide disaster has been a huge lesson to the world which shocked the entire health care teams. On analyzing the disaster, it was found that new drugs were introduced into the market in haste without proper scientific studies after administration to human beings. Hence, the process of introducing new drugs was lengthened and tightened. Also, it was found that generally there is no one to monitor the effects of drugs, especially the adverse reactions of a drug on the human body after administration. Hence, the concept of clinical pharmacy was evolved, in which the pharmacist is given the responsibility of doing Therapeutic Drug Monitoring (TDM) i.e., monitoring the drug's action after administration to the patients.

Also, the concept of clinical pharmacy is helpful in assuaging the feelings of common people who were not only angry but also reluctant to go to an allopathic doctor for treatment or take allopathic drugs after the Thalidomide tragedy. They started looking for alternative systems of medicine and from then onwards, herbal drugs gained popularity. Hence, the concept of clinical pharmacy gives the assurance that people's welfare after administering the drugs will be looked after by an expert, the Clinical Pharmacist, by regular monitoring and intervention in case of something going wrong. Thus, the old pattern of treatment "diagnosing, writing a prescription, dispensing drugs and forgetting the patient" was put to an end by this concept. The need for clinical pharmacy services is, thus, crystal clear.

DEFINITION

Clinical pharmacy is defined as a system concerned with rational selection and use of medicaments at the patient level so as to ensure the patient's maximum well being while on drug therapy.

Basis of Clinical Pharmacy

Because of the nature of their job, clinical pharmacists have to be in continuous touch with the medical professional and also the details of the treatment of the patients. Hence, apart from the usual pharmacy subjects, they have to be familiar with Biochemistry, Clinical Pathology, Pathophysiology, etc. That is why these subjects were introduced into the diploma and degree syllabus of pharmacy. They must be thorough with subjects such as Biopharmaceutics, Pharmacokinetics, and Pharmacodynamics which are the basis for clinical pharmacy.

While Biopharmaceutics deals with bioavailability, dosage regimen, and different formulations, Pharmacokinetics deals with the significance of absorption, distribution, metabolism, and excretion of drugs. Pharmacodynamics, on the other hand, describes the effect of drugs on the body. These subjects lay the foundation for clinical pharmacy.

Needless to mention, the knowledge of chemical analysis of body fluids and other samples for drugs is very essential in determining or adjusting the dose for individual patients, which is considered to be a primary duty of a clinical pharmacist. Thus, all the above subjects, hitherto neglected by pharmacists, form the basis of clinical pharmacy.

Functions of Clinical Pharmacist

It is safe to conclude that a clinical pharmacist has a multidimensional role. Few of them are routine, others are rare and the remaining yet need specialization. Thus, a clinical pharmacist has to perform the following duties routinely:

1. Getting a patient's medication history

2. Offering consultation to physicians in the selection of suitable drug for the particular patient or selecting the drugs themselves

3. Therapeutic drug monitoring including body fluid analysis and

4. Counseling the patients.

Apart from these regular functions, a clinical pharmacist may be assigned some specific duties when needed. For example, they have to detect and confirm suspected Adverse Drug Reactions [ADR] occurred in a particular patient. Similarly, they may be required to prepare

Total Parenteral Nutrition (TPN) for some patients. Though these works are not required to be performed often, they are assigned to senior Clinical Pharmacists, nevertheless.

In big tertiary care hospitals, complicated and referral cases may require some degree of specialization to attend. Thus, pediatric, geriatric and psychiatric cases need specialization. Also, a clinical pharmacist's specialized services are required in difficult situations such as narcotic withdrawal treatment, the study of clinical toxicology, and complicated pharmacokinetic studies.

Routine and General Functions

1. **Medication history interview:** Immediately after admitting the patient into the ward, the diagnostic tests begin and the medication history of the patient has to be obtained. Because pharmacists are mostly involved in providing drugs to the patient both in hospital pharmacy and outside community pharmacy, they can get a comprehensive medication history from the patient. A pharmacist is more suitable for this job than anybody else in the health care team. They have to get the drug history involving prescription drugs, and self-medication and OTC drugs. We will discuss the art of obtaining useful medication history in detail later.

2. **Offering consultation for drug selection:** Because of the stiff competition among the pharmaceutical companies to market their products, doctors are supplied with either biased information or half-truth about a particular formulation. As a busy doctor has no time to verify the authenticity of that information, a clinical pharmacist can be of great help. They are able to deliver an unbiased report about the usefulness of a particular drug on a particular patient in a particular condition. They are experts on drugs and drug information. Their main task is to ensure the rational and safe use of the drug. So, they are in a better position to correct the deficiencies in the use of drugs by patients and doctors alike.

   The ward where the clinical pharmacist is posted has all the information available about the patient. This makes them able to advise on the best formulation to suit the particular patient needs. Similarly, they can discourage the use of unnecessary drugs more effectively whilst on the ward than from the dispensary where the relevant background information is not usually available. Alternatively, if the authorities agree, they can select the drug on their own and write the prescription, as practiced in the USA.

3. **Therapeutic drug monitoring and analysis of body fluids:** As mentioned earlier, the clinical pharmacist is mainly appointed to monitor the patients after the administration of drugs. To do that effectively, they have to undertake plasma/blood drug concentration studies. The blood samples at regular intervals are collected from the patient and then analyzed. These results help the pharmacist to arrive at a suitable dose for the particular patient. Also, it helps them in assessing the usefulness of drug on that particular patient, so that they can suggest the doctor to either increase or decrease the dose or stop it altogether and go for an alternative.

   The clinical pharmacists are able to do this because they not only have the knowledge of pharmacological properties of a drug but also their physical, chemical and pharmaceutical properties. This is something that is not taught to doctors. Hence, clinical pharmacists are able to predict the possible adverse effects, any drug interaction possibilities, and any other factor which can modify the drug activity. Their attention is mainly drawn to the drugs with narrow therapeutic indices and requires careful dose adjustment in the event of predisposing factors like old age, renal failure, hepatic damage, and concurrent medication. Thus, a clinical pharmacist is able to contribute significantly to direct patient care by performing TDM.

4. **Patient counseling:** Counselling is nothing but advising and convincing the patient about drug therapy. As a result of counseling, patient compliance with the instructions improves. Making the patients realize that their disease can be cured if they adhere to certain instructions can help the health care team deliver successful treatment results. With effective counseling, the patients stop complaining about the bitter tablets, frequent pricks, and painful lab procedures. They gradually realize that everything is done is in favor of their well-being. Counseling is done during the treatment and also at the time of discharge regarding the dos and don'ts after the discharge. Thus, patient counseling is considered as a major function of a clinical pharmacist.

Specific Functions

5. **Detection of adverse drug reactions:** It is only possible through the monitoring of the patient, closely and continuously. As therapeutic drug monitoring (TDM) is one of the main duties of clinical pharmacists, they are in a better position to detect the Adverse Drug Reactions (ADR). These occur infrequently or only after a prolonged administration of the drug, and hence, they can only be detected among inpatients of the hospital and not outpatients. There are a few exceptions like chronic cases of diabetics, hypertension, etc.

Since it is very unlikely to detect the ADR during pre-marketing studies, a Clinical Pharmacist's service in this area is considered important and invaluable. Once such ADR is detected, it is fully investigated to ascertain its frequency and distribution. This information is then passed on to authorities concerned (like National Pharmacovigilance centers, WHO, Drugs Control Department, etc) who, in turn, pass it on to the medical profession, pharmaceutical manufacturers and others.

6. **Total Parenteral Nutrition:** This is also a specific and particular patient-oriented service that a clinical pharmacist can provide. They may be assigned the task of formulating and preparing the Total Parenteral Nutrition (TPN) for a particular patient who may not be in a position to take food via the oral route. The clinical pharmacist can take the need for a particular mineral or vitamin into account as they are aware of the drug regimen and deficiencies of the particular patient. Thus, they can be of much help to prescribers and nurses in providing better treatment to the patient.

Special Functions

Similar to medical specialties, a clinical pharmacist can also specialize in certain areas of practice. For example, treatment to the following patients need careful attention and monitoring, and hence, specialization:

(a) Pediatric cases
(b) Geriatric cases
(c) Psychiatric cases and
(d) Drug addiction cases

As the pharmacokinetics and consequently the pharmacodynamics of the drugs administered to these categories of patients differ from normal adult patients, a careful selection of drug, its dose, and monitoring are needed. For example, in the case of Narcotic withdrawal treatment, a correct dose needs to be administered to control the episodes of violence, seizures, etc. Hence, a clinical pharmacist needs to specialize in these areas too and help the medical profession in treating these risky cases. Also, they may have to specialize in clinical toxicology and poison cases in order to improve the safe and rational use of drugs and save lives.

Functions of a Clinical Pharmacist

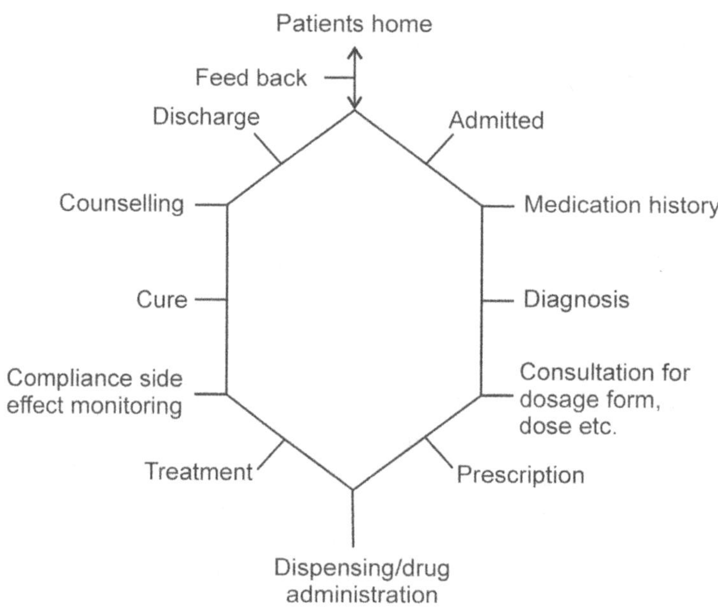

Fig. 17.1 Sides of hexagon: Existing functions of a hospital (without Clinical Pharmacist) Joints of sides of hexagon: Functions of a Clinical Pharmacist

Skills required for a Clinical Pharmacist

In order to perform the functions discussed above, a clinical pharmacist needs to develop and acquire many skills and talents. For example, to obtain a useful and thorough medication history, they need to have good communication and convincing abilities. As they are going to discuss the patient's personal life during the medication history interview, the answers may not include complete facts. The pharmacist must be able to develop a rapport with patients by making them realize that they are working for the patient's welfare. Such a rapport, if developed, will lead to a successful medication interview. They need to have the ability to put clever questions without hurting the feelings of the patient to get the correct and complete answer.

Similarly, to offer consultation to the treating physician who already has a fair knowledge of drugs and formulations, its dose and uses, a clinical pharmacist needs to know over and above what a physician has. Hence, a thorough, up to date and full knowledge of drugs, therapeutics, and problems with particular drugs are essential. They should be able to provide this information on the spot, without referring to books and other sources. Thus, very good subject knowledge is a must for a clinical pharmacist.

Therapeutic Drug Monitoring (TDM) requires keen observation of the patients for the progress in treatment as well as for signs and symptoms of Adverse Drug Reactions. Once identified, they must be able to establish ADR by necessary tests and analysis. Analyzing body fluids and other samples is very difficult because the samples are collected from a living, dynamic human body. It has many variations and interferences and so, it requires sound analytical skills.

The counseling of patients, again, points to the need for effective communication. It also requires empathy, patience, and convincing skills. All the patients' doubts must be cleared and the clinical pharmacist must make them understand the need for adhering to instructions. Thereby, compliance and consequently, the outcome of the treatment is highly improved.

Once these basic skills are acquired by education and experience, the clinical pharmacists need to specialize in their areas of interest or requirement. They must able to do research in the area of specialization and acquire wide and in-depth knowledge in that field. They should also publish research papers in reputed journals and conferences. This will help the clinical pharmacist become of the most important links in the health care team.

DRUG THERAPY MONITORING

DEFINITION

Drug therapy monitoring or review is a process by which a clinical pharmacist reviews the patient's treatment regimen to ensure effective, safe and economical therapy.

Needless to say, it is the responsibility of the clinical pharmacist to ensure the best therapy possible for each patient. To do that effectively, a clinical pharmacist must be knowledgeable in pharmacokinetics, pharmacodynamics, therapeutics, ADR, lab data analysis, and clinical reasoning. All these require information from various sources and they must be able to interpret and utilize them properly. They should carry out this review daily for complicated cases and periodically for other cases. They must be ready with this review before participating in ward round along with treating physicians.

Purpose of Drug Therapy Monitoring (DTM)

The prime purpose of DTM is effective, safe and economical therapy for all patients.

However, by undertaking DTM a clinical pharmacist is able to identify

(a) Patients who are in need of counseling

(b) Patients who require special attention and

(c) Patients with the risk of medication error.

To achieve these purposes, the DTR must be broad-based and multi-component in nature. They are discussed below:

Scope of DTM

Drug Therapy Monitoring or Review (DTR) is a broad function of a domain of which the Therapeutic Drug Monitoring (TDM) is one of the components. In order to perform DTR, the clinical pharmacist needs to prepare beforehand. DTR is actually the review of the entire therapy of patients with drugs. Hence, to arrive at a correct conclusion, the clinical pharmacist should know the previous and present condition of the patient. They have to assess the treatment goals, and how far and how best it is achievable. They must be sure whether the present therapy is proceeding on the correct line to achieve the set goal.

It may not be easy for complicated cases and sometimes even more difficult for cases with manageable problems as there are chances of patients developing complications during the course of treatment. For example, there could be drug-related problems like non-responsiveness to the standard drug regimen, sub-therapeutic dose, over dosage, adverse drug reactions including drug-drug interaction, drug-food interaction or drug-disease interaction.

Hence, therapeutic drug monitoring (TDM) by body fluid analysis or pharmacokinetic studies should be carried out wherever necessary. Using the data obtained from TDM, the dose of the drug should be individualized to arrive at a correct regimen.

Thereafter, the therapy must be monitored closely in order to find out treatment outcomes. Thus, the scope of DTR extends from patient medication history to TDM and beyond.

Duties Involved in DTR

As indicated above, the first and foremost duty involved in DTR is collecting as much information as possible about the patient's previous and present condition. This includes collecting information about patients' past medical history including prevailing diseases before present illness and treatment undertaken or undergoing, allergy or sensitivity to drugs, habits, daily routines, etc. Along with the above details, present condition, treatment, and clinical progress or otherwise will lay the foundation for drug therapy review.

This information can be gathered from various sources like the patient's medication history interview, laboratory results, nursing notes, observational charts, and case sheets. As described elsewhere in this book, the value of a medication history interview is well-known. It not only reveals almost everything about the patient's present and past problems but also helps in finding etiology or reasons for the present problem and for arriving at a correct diagnosis and drug regimen. An interview conducted by a clinical pharmacist can also reveal the drugs already used by the patient, especially the OTC drugs, drugs from alternative systems of medicine, household remedies, etc.

The next important duty in DTR is setting and evaluating the treatment target. The complete cure is what patients want but that may not be possible every time. Hence, a realistic target must be fixed like the reduction of severity of the disease, elimination of the symptoms of the disease, slowing the advancement of the disease, etc. The treatment goals are patient-specific and differ from patient to patient due to the factors like age, weakness or susceptibility, etc. This goal of therapy should be reviewed periodically and the progress must be evaluated. Furthermore, suitable corrections are made and then the reasons for failure are analyzed. For this, the entire team involved in the treatment of the particular patient is consulted and involved actively in the correction process.

Another crucial duty in DTR is the identification of drug-related problems that occurred during the present therapy. If the treatment is in a hospital where clinical pharmacist's services are available, problems like inappropriate drug selection, sub-therapeutic dose or over dosages are less. However, even these problems may occur in a few cases, hence, a quick review must be carried out during DTR. More series problems like complications due to untreated indications, patient's multiple diseases, organ failures, adverse drug reactions occurred during the course of treatment, etc. have to be reviewed carefully.

Once the drug-related problems, if any, is identified and resolved, the next step is to correct the regimen to suit the individual patient. This can be achieved by switching over to sustained release, once a day formulations, changing the route of administration, time of administrations, etc. While changing the regimen to suit the individual, the cost-effectiveness of the therapy must be taken into consideration while also ensuring the compliance of the regimen by the patient. Multiple drug prescriptions or polypharmacy must be controlled as much as possible by including combination drugs, wherever possible.

After carrying out all the duties during DTR, the results of the treatment must be monitored. For this, the clinical review and tests carried out by and on the instructions of the treating physician are highly useful. The laboratory data such as the results of blood tests, x-ray, scan, liver function tests, kidney function tests, etc. can be used for the purpose of monitoring. Some drugs may produce the desired results after a fairly long time. For example, antidepressants require 30 to 40 days to produce a response in patients. However, if a drug does not produce the required result within a reasonable time, a careful review of the drug prescribed must be made. There could be a requirement of increasing the dose or replacing the drug with some other drug or addition of one more drug to the regimen.

Medication Chart Review

This is one of the most important duties assigned to clinical pharmacists in developed countries, in order to prevent medication errors and to ensure the best treatment possible for the patients. It has become an essential function in these countries because patients sue the doctors and hospitals for a very huge sum as compensation in the courts if anything goes wrong during the course of the treatment. A scenario like this does not exist in our country yet but we are slowly picking up. Here, the medication chart review is yet to be implemented. However, the future pharmacists need to know the process of reviewing the medication chart as these duties will also be assigned in India, sooner or later. Medication errors are preventable errors that may occur during prescription writing and drug administration. To prevent these errors, pharmacists must systematically review the medication charts. The following are the guidelines to carry out medication chart review:

1. Poorly written, illegible prescriptions should be returned to the prescriber and checked. There should be no guess-work involved in the process.

2. The identity of the patient must be clear, for which the name, age, sex, hospital number of the patient should be clearly written on the medication chart. If not, check and write.

3. If the patient is allergic to some drugs or tests, it should be legibly written in the space provided in the medication chart with red ink. If no allergies are identified, it should also be mentioned in that place too.

4. The name of the drug, dose, and route of administration should be written by the treating physician and it should be checked. No abbreviations should be used to write the name of the drug. As much as possible, generic names should be written on the chart. If not, the pharmacist should write it, next to the brand name. The dose and dosage interval should be correct and as intended by the doctor, depending on the patient's condition. Any unusual dose should be underlined by him, to indicate he mean it. Decimals should be avoided as far as possible as they may lead to ten times more dose, if not seen properly. For example, it should be 5 mg, not 5.0 mg and 0.5 gm, not .5 gm.

5. The time of administration should also be mentioned in the medication chart. If it is not suitable for the particular patient, like there is a possibility of drug-drug interaction or drug-food interaction, the pharmacist can write annotation on the chart, recommending a change in time of administration of the particular drug.

6. The prescriptions with instructions like SOS (whenever necessary) should have minimum dose interval to adhere, otherwise, there is a possibility of over dosage.

7. Additional instructions like after food, before food, with plenty of water, etc., can be written by the clinical pharmacist wherever necessary.

8. The medications should be prescribed according to the legal and local requirements of the government concerned. It should be signed and dated by the prescriber and any corrections in the medication chart should be endorsed by them.

9. The medication chart should also be signed by the nurse who administers the drug to the patient, in the space provided. Thus, the medication chart will be a complete and authentic record of the treatment given to the patient.

Model Mediation Chart XYZ Hospital

Patient name: .... IP No: .... Unit: ....

Age: .... Sex: .... Height: .... Weight: ....

Allergy:..

S. No.	Name of the drug	Dose	Route	Time of admn.	Day of administration (Nurse initials)							
					1st	2nd	3rd	4th	5th	6th	7th	8th
1.				8am 2pm 8pm								
	Additional instructions											
	Signature of doctor with date											
2.												
	Additional instructions											
	Signature of doctor with date											
3.												
	Additional instructions											
	Signature of doctor with date											
4.												
	Additional instructions											
	Signature of doctor with date											
5.												
	Additional instructions											
	Signature of doctor with date											

CLINICAL REVIEW AND PHARMACIST INTERVENTION

Need for Clinical Review

There are a lot of variables among the patients like age, weight, sex, disease and its severity, body mass, genetic makeup, kidney damage, liver damage, concurrently administered drugs, and the environment. All these variables affect the effect of the drug on a particular individual. Hence, a common dose or a dose guessed to be suitable cannot be expected to produce the desired effect. This is a major problem of any therapy, however, it is ignored in short time therapies like the one given to outpatients of the hospitals, who are treated for short term illness. But for the patients who require prolonged therapy, this problem cannot be set aside. Among the variables listed above, co-administration of many drugs to patient causes problems. We can predict the action of one drug given alone to a patient but if two or more drugs are administered to a patient at the same time, there will be unexpected effects. For example, ketoconazole, an antifungal, potentiate the effect of cyclosporine-- an immunosuppressant. Thus, the pharmacokinetic and the pharmacodynamic properties of one drug are affected by a completely unrelated drug, if given together.

Thus, a normal dose of a drug may produce a normal effect in some patients, a toxic effect in some other patients, and altogether ineffective in yet another patient. Hence, the need for optimizing the dose for an individual is evident.

There are some drugs that have a narrow therapeutic index. Hence, there is a danger of a toxic effect to the patient if the dose is not proper. Similarly, some drugs produce huge effects even for a small change in dose and some other drugs that are critically needed for therapy, though dangerous to use in a given situation, are used with probable risks involved. For all these drugs, a dose suitable for the individual patient should be calculated and used. Examples for these drugs are digoxin, phenytoin, theophylline, and cyclosporine.

Parameters Useful in Clinical Review and Individualization of Dose

The following are the important parameters, otherwise known as pharmacokinetic data useful in the individualization of dosage regimen:

1. Bioavailability
2. Protein binding
3. Volume of distribution
4. Clearance and
5. Half-life

The clinical pharmacist must be thorough with all these parameters and should be able to calculate them accurately by performing necessary tests on the individual patient. They should be able to correlate and interpret these data and arrive at the correct dose by necessary calculations.

The above parameters are explained below in detail.

1. **Bioavailability:** After an oral dose, a certain percentage of that drug reaches the systematic circulation and produces a therapeutic effect. This fraction or percentage of the drug is known as the bioavailability of that particular drug.

   The entire drug administered is not absorbed into the circulation. A part of it is inactivated in the GI mucosa or metabolized by the liver (First pass metabolism) and only the remaining percentage is available for pharmacological action. This is due to several factors given below:

   (i)   **Factors that affect absorption:** If the absorption of the drug is affected, it naturally affects the bioavailability. Hence, factors like solubility of a particular drug, its physical-chemical properties, the concentration of the drug, surface area of absorption, circulation to the site of absorption, presence of food or water in the stomach, etc affect bioavailability.

   (ii) Anatomical site from which the drug is absorbed also has an important role to play in bioavailability. For example, if taken by the oral route, it is first metabolized in the liver and excreted in the bile, hence, the bioavailability is altered.

   (iii) Diseases that alter the structure and function of the GI tract also affect the bioavailability.

2. **Protein Binding:** All drugs are bound to plasma and/or tissue proteins to some extent. Protein binding is the percentage of drug that is bound to plasma protein to the concentration of drug in the blood. If something disturbs the protein binding of a drug, then more drugs may be freely circulating in the plasma. As we know that only the free drug concentration is responsible for pharmacological action, this phenomenon should be monitored. A change in protein binding also alters the distribution and excretion of the drug. Hence, before attempting to individualize the therapy of a patient, this factor should be considered seriously.

3. **Volume of Distribution (Vd):** It is the total fluid volume required for the dose of the drug given to the patient to be distributed throughout the body at the same concentration as in plasma. But it is not as simple. It requires a detailed explanation, starting from the administration of an oral dose. The dose of the drug given to the patient is distributed in the body through the vascular system. Majority of the drugs have sufficient lipophilicity and hence, they are able to distribute both in the intra and extracellular compartments of the body. Thus, the drug reaches to tissues and the process is called distribution.

   The volume of distribution as mentioned above is not an identifiable physiological volume but an imaginary volume that is required to distribute the given drug at the same concentration as in the blood or plasma.

If we take the body as a single compartment, the body fluids are:

Blood volume: 5.5 L

Plasma volume   :   3.0 L

Extracellular fluid   :   12.0 L

Total body water   :   42.0L

The distribution of the drug may be in the blood, extracellular fluid, or into the tissue. The drugs that are distributed only in the blood will have the volume of distribution close to blood volume 5.5 L. For example, the volume of distribution (Vd) of Furosemide is 7.7L. Similarly, drugs that reach extracellular space but not the tissue will have a Vd of around 20 L. e.g.: Atenolol, Theophylline, etc (Vd = 20 to 40 L) and drugs that enter tissues will have a still larger volume of distribution.

e.g.: Vd of chloroquine = 13,000 L; Digoxin = 700 L

This unrealistic value is obtained because of this drug's low concentration in blood (and the majority of the drug distributed up to tissue). The volume of distribution of a drug is calculated by the following formulae:

$$V_d = \frac{f_D}{C_p} \quad \text{[For oral dose]}$$

where f is the fraction of drug available (Bioavailability) D is the amount of drug given (Dose)

Cp is the concentration in plasma

$$V_d \text{ (For Inj)} = \frac{\text{Total injected drug}}{\text{Plasma conc.}}$$

4. **Clearance:** It is the volume of plasma freed of the drug per minute. The organs of clearance are kidney and liver. However, it also takes place at other places like in sweat, saliva, bile, stomach, fecal loss, loss in lungs and at other sites of metabolism. Total systemic clearance is obtained by adding all these separate clearances.

CL Renal + CL Hepatic + CL Others = CL Systemic

Clearances by main organs like kidney or liver are calculated by the following formula:

$$C_{LR} \text{ (Renal clearance)} = \frac{UV}{P}$$

where

U is the concentration of drug in urine

V is the average volume of urine/minute

P is the concentration of drug in plasma

$$C_{LH} \text{ (Hepatic clearance)} = \frac{Q \times (C_{in} - C_{out})}{C_{in}}$$

Where Q: Blood Flow

C_{in}: Concentration of drug going into the liver

C_{out}: Concentration of drug coming out of the liver

Clearance can also be calculated by another formula

$$CL = \frac{V_d}{t_{1/2}}$$

where Vd is the volume of distribution,

$t_{1/2}$ is half life

If clearance is more, naturally, the half-life will be less. Only when the fractional availability of the drug is known, clearance can be calculated. Hence, to accurately calculate the clearance, the oral dose is not reliable, and therefore, it is determined following I.V dosage where the availability is 100% of the dose given.

Use or Value of Studying Clearance

The plasma concentration of drugs keeps varying due to various factors. But the physician wants to keep a steady-state concentration of drugs in the patient's plasma, so as to achieve the goals of the treatment. This can be achieved only when the rate of elimination is equal to the rate of administration of the drug. Simply put, the input should be equal to output. i.e.,

The dosing rate = CL. Css, where CL is clearance and Css, is the steady-state concentration of the drug.

Thus, if we know the desired steady-state concentration of the drug, the clearance dictates the rate at which the drug should be administered. Then, the maintenance dose and dosing interval can be determined. The study of clearance is also very useful in clinical pharmacokinetics as it is constant over a range of dose and consequent plasma concentrations.

2. **Half-life:** Half-life can be defined as the time taken by the body to eliminate half of the amount of the drug in the body. The following table is self-explanatory.

At the end of	Plasma Conc. in mg	Total Drug Eliminated
0 Time	100	NIL
1st Half life	50	50%
2nd Half life	25	75%
3rd Half life	12.5	87.5%
4th Half life	6.25	93.75%
5th Half life	3.125	96.875%

Thus, after the 5th Half-life, almost all the drug is removed from the body. To compare the pharmacokinetics of a drug in a normal person and diseased patient, this parameter is very useful.

Alteration of the Pharmacokinetic Parameters in the Individual Patient which require Attention and Intervention by Pharmacist

Pharmacokinetic parameters that are discussed above are altered or determined by many physiological and biochemical events that occur in normal people and the pathological conditions that may exist only in a particular disease. Hence, a clinical pharmacist must be thorough with those conditions and intervene when necessary.

I. Bioavailability

The following factors affect the bioavailability of a drug that requires monitoring by the pharmacist.

1. Patient's non-compliance to the drug regimen
2. Poor formulations like tablets with less solubility
3. Drug-Drug Interactions
4. Drug-Food Interactions
5. Metabolism of a drug in GI Tract
6. First pass metabolism by the liver
7. Biliary excretion
8. Poor Metabolism of certain drugs by the liver (e.g., Lidocaine)
9. The surface area of absorption
10. Pathological conditions of the stomach
11. Physical and chemical properties of the drug and
12. Amount or concentration of drug in the GI tract

As so many factors affect the bioavailability, frequent checking of this parameter helps in continuation or modification of the drug regimen.

II. Protein binding

Protein binding is mainly affected by liver damage which, in turn, affects the production of albumin and other proteins. If the nitrogenous waste materials are not properly removed from the body, then also the protein binding is affected (the condition is called Uraemia). Once protein binding is affected, it leads to huge changes in the volume of distribution due to increase in free-drug concentration or binding of drugs in tissue proteins.

III. Volume of distribution

The following factors affect the volume of distribution:

1. pka of the drug (Log of the dissociation constant of a weak acid)
2. Degree of binding to plasma proteins
3. The partition coefficient of the drug in fat
4. Degree of binding to tissue proteins
5. Patient's age, sex, and body composition and
6. The disease of the patient

If the plasma concentration is very low and when the fraction of the drug available in the body is divided by it, a huge volume of distribution is obtained. Sometimes, it may be thousands of liters as in the case of chloroquine and hence, highly unrealistic. However, the volume of distribution thus obtained is also useful as it indicates the extent of binding of the drug to the tissue protein. This knowledge is again very helpful in the treatment of drug overdose cases when any amount of hemodialysis or haemoperfusion will not be useful as that will reduce plasma concentration only temporarily and the drug will redistribute from tissue to plasma after the dialysis. Thus, alternative methods of treatment should be given to the patient as quickly as possible.

IV.   Clearance

The following factors alter the clearance of a drug by an organ

1. Blood flow to the organ
2. The fraction of the drug unbound in the blood (free drug concentration) and
3. The ability of the organ to remove the free drug

If any of the above factors are affected due to disease, the clearance is altered. Thus, liver damage and kidney damage play an important role in clearance.

V.   Half-Life

Though half-life does not depend on the body mass of the patient, indirectly, it is affected because it depends on the volume of distribution which is proportional to the body size. If the clearance decreases due to disease, half-life increases. Similarly, if the volume of distribution is reduced due to age (less body mass), clearance is increased and consequently the half-life is affected. Thus, these problems start from the number of proteins available for binding by a drug, and continue to affect the volume of distribution, clearance, and finally the half-life. These parameters are thus interdependent and well-connected with each other and hence, should not be viewed in isolation.

Pharmacodynamic Parameters

The parameters described above are all pharmacokinetic, depending on the absorption, distribution, metabolism, and excretion (ADME) of the drug. However, there are other parameters that affect the pharmacodynamics of the drug. Pharmacodynamic is the study of the effects of the drug on the body. While pharmacokinetics describes "what the body does to the drug, pharmacodynamic deals with "what the drug does to the body".

For many drugs, the effect cannot be quantified. Similarly, the amount of drug required to produce a certain effect on the site of action is also difficult to estimate. It is because there is little or negligible information about the receptor number, drug affinity, subsequent coupling of drug with the receptor, or the effect of disease on these factors, etc. Hence, the relationship between the effect and plasma concentration is unknown. This relationship is very complicated and disturbed by many factors. For example, the effective concentration of an antibiotic depends not only on the dose but also on the type of microorganisms. Apart from it, the drug effect is ultimately affected by the pharmacokinetic factors. Hence, if we want to correlate both pharmacokinetic and pharmacodynamic factors, the time of distribution of the drug to the site of action must also be taken into account. All these make the study complicated.

Pharmacist's Intervention

The clinical pharmacist has to adjust all mean parameters for individual patients carefully. To calculate the desired steady-state concentration of a drug, free drug circulation in the blood (bioavailability) should be known. To arrive at the maintenance dose, a fraction of the drug absorbed and clearance must be estimated. To compute the loading dose and to estimate half-life and dosing interval, the volume of distribution is needed. Thus, bioavailability, clearance, and volume of distribution are important parameters in adjusting or individualizing the dose for a patient, which a clinical pharmacist must keep in mind while intervening in therapy.

WARD ROUND PARTICIPATION

INTRODUCTION

A ward round is when a medical practitioner goes around the ward of the hospital where the patients are admitted for review or follow up of the treatment given to each patient. This is done by them either alone or along with junior doctors and other members of the health care team. This is undertaken either daily or at fixed time intervals, depending on the need and rules of the hospital.

Usually, only chief or senior doctors go on a ward round with their assistant doctors, house surgeons or interns and medical students. The assistant doctors who are actually involved in treating the patients get advice and suggestions from the senior or chief doctor regarding the treatment and make multiple visits to the ward on a single day with or without somebody accompanying them.

Thus, the chief doctor's visit to the ward acquires significance when the entire health care team is available for taking instructions and for consultation.

Ward Rounds and Pharmacists

Until recently and even today in many countries including India, pharmacists are not included in ward rounds. In the developed Western countries, after the 1970s, the clinical pharmacists were asked to participate in ward rounds as the value of their services was acknowledged by then. During ward rounds, the clinical pharmacists provide valuable information to the doctors on different formulations, their strength, availability, side effects, suitability for the particular patient, alternative or substitute drugs, etc, on the spot. That is to say, that the information is given when it is needed the most, that is, at the time of prescription writing for the inpatients. Thus, they help the medical practitioner to ensure the safe and rational use of drugs and thereby, achieving improved patient care at less cost and time.

Types of Ward Rounds

There are many types of ward rounds, depending on the purpose and the person. Though chief doctor of the ward undertakes authoritative, decision making ward rounds, prior to that, other members of the health care team also make ward rounds for definite purposes. For example, house surgeons or P.G Medical students go on a preliminary ward round to prepare and get ready for chief doctors round. They collect the required information about each patient and the outcome of the previous round's decisions. For instance, they collect lab results for tests prescribed for the patient on the previous round and keep ready the summary of it for the chief doctor's attention. The clinical pharmacist can also undertake such preliminary round and be ready with drug-related information.

The second type of ward round is by Resident Medical Officer [RMO], who is in- charge of the overall activities of the hospital. Most of the time, their rounds will be of administrative in nature and outside of the actual treatment of the patient. Nevertheless, they enquire the patient or the healthcare team about the patient's grievances or discomfort, if any, for the purpose of rectifying the same. They are accompanied by assistant doctors, interns, and nurses. These visits are not undertaken daily but a few times in a month.

The third type of important ward round is by the chief doctor of the ward or the department. They review the previous round's decisions and their results and give instructions about the further course of treatment to the patient while the team makes a note of it. Most of the time, the chief doctor explains the clinical aspects including diagnosis, symptoms, disease manifestations, treatment, and its outcome during this visit to house surgeons and medical students who take note of all these things while at the bedside of the patient. The clinical pharmacist can also use these briefings to further improve their clinical knowledge.

The fourth type of ward round is by the academic staff of teaching hospitals. The associate or assistant professors of the medical, surgical or other departments of medical colleges visit for the purpose of teaching their students about relevant cases admitted in the wards. After a brief lecture-demonstration of the cases, follow-up classes on a particular topic or disease are held in the classrooms available in the hospital itself or in their colleges. This ensures that the students acquire practical knowledge of the subject. Most of the time, clinical pharmacists have no role in this round.

Preparation for Ward Round by Clinical Pharmacist

A clinical pharmacist needs to be prepared for the ward round by the chief doctor of the ward. They may have to offer consultation regarding the medicines prescribed for the inpatients of the ward. For this purpose, they may need to prepare the following:

1. Medication profile of each patient
2. Summary of a medication history of each patient
3. Summary of a Drug Utilization review
4. The recommendation they indents to make based on the above documents and
5. Supportive documents and references for the above.

In spite of the best care by the entire health care team, there is still a possibility for drug interaction, adverse drug reaction, and medication error. Drug-Diet interaction, Drug-Diagnostic test interaction, Drug-Disease interaction are the three DDs that a clinical pharmacist needs to watch. The other types of reactions are mostly avoided by the treating team through careful planning and monitoring.

A model form of Patient Medication Profile is given below. With slight variations, they are maintained in all the hospitals where clinical pharmacy services are available. A clinical pharmacist has to keep it updated and ready for ward rounds.

During the discussion for the selection of drugs for the patients, their medication history is very useful. The treating clinician must at least possess its summary if the full history is not available for reference. The history is not only useful while prescribing immediately after diagnosis but also during the course of treatment, depending on the patient's response or otherwise for the drugs administered. This factor makes it an important document until the patient's discharge.

If Drug Utilization Evaluation [DUE] has been undertaken on the particular patient by the DUE team and its report is communicated to the treating team, the clinical pharmacist must be ready with a copy of it. It helps in course correction in the light of recommendations made by the DUE team.

Finally, a clinical pharmacist should prepare a document on their intentions to make any recommendation to change a drug or its dose or addition of another drug, etc. They should be able to cite relevant references for their recommendations so that the treating clinical practitioner accepts it without any hesitation.

All the above groundwork by the clinical pharmacists ensures better treatment for the patient and appreciation for their services.

Pharmacist Interventions

There are many contributions and a few interventions that a clinical pharmacist has to make during ward rounds. The clinical pharmacists have limitations like they only have authority on drugs and related matters. Hence, as much as possible, they should not interfere with the diagnosis, pathology, and etiology of diseases. However, this does not mean they should not raise their concerns over the toxic effect manifestations of the drug on the patient. They should be vigilant while watching for ADR or drug interactions and report the observations to the treating clinician.

In many hospitals where clinical pharmacy services are fully established, they are empowered to order investigative lab tests to confirm the drug's toxicity. If the results of these tests confirm the suspicion, they can boldly intervene in the treatment process equipped with test results from the lab. Thus, a clinical pharmacist's intervention should be, as much as possible, based on solid evidence. Subsequently, such interventions are appreciated by the health care team. After gaining the confidence of the chief doctor and the team in this way, their future doubts and observations will be given due attention even before the lab results.

Pharmacist's Contribution during Ward Rounds

Most of the times, a clinical pharmacist's contribution during ward rounds will be on matters relating to drugs. Doctors, nurses and medical students may require the following information on the spot:

1. Formulations [Dosage forms]

2. Dose

3. Indications and contraindications

4. Drugs availability and its supply source

5. Economy [price]

6. Substitute [if the above is not available]

7. The time required for getting the supply

8. Legal and administrative issues and

9. Special storage conditions, if any.

If the clinical pharmacist is able to give this information immediately, without referring to any book or source of information, their value and respect among the team peaks and a fruitful team spirit develops. This results in adding to the reputation of the hospital.

Limitations of Ward Rounds

A chief doctor is always hard-pressed for time to undertake elaborate ward rounds. Their services are required in situations like emergency cases, on sudden complications developed in existing cases and in administrative matters. Hence, he tries to make ward rounds short and useful. The clinical pharmacists need to understand this and present their recommendations and suggestions short and precise to the point. If it is evident that less time is available for ward-round, they should intervene in cases that are more important and require immediate attention. Other cases can wait till next ward round.

If there is no fixed time for ward-rounds in a hospital, they should make arrangements to get prior intimation about the time of ward rounds. In some hospitals, the clinical pharmacist has to look after more than one ward at the same time. If simultaneous ward rounds are going on certain wards, the clinical pharmacist has to prioritize patients based on the need of the intervention and then attend the ward round where the particular patient is present. For the patients in another ward, they can make annotations in the medication chart, if the hospital pharmacy permits it.

The drug therapy review requires medication chart endorsement by a clinical pharmacist in order to ensure that prescriptions are unambiguous, clear and legible without any doubt. Hence, clinical pharmacists are permitted to make annotations in prescriptions in hospitals where clinical pharmacy services are fully organized. However, face to face discussions among the health care team members ensure better coordination in the treatment process. But it may not be always possible due to various reasons. Some suggestions may not be acceptable to one or the other members of the team and might need elaborate discussions. This can not be done by standing by the side of the patient. The team may meet in the cabin of ward doctor or someplace else. After thorough discussions, correct decisions are made by reviewing material facts and then they are properly implemented. If the situation requires no immediate decision, the team can call for additional information or evidence. Until its availability, the decision can be postponed. Thus, the ward round has its own limitations and the pharmacists should learn to perform their duties within these limitations.

Skills Needed for Ward Round Participation

In order to communicate with the multidisciplinary team of the ward round, the clinical pharmacist needs to acquire two important skills: clinical knowledge and communication talent. To develop clinical knowledge, the pharmacists first need to understand and use the clinical terms. Depending upon the ward where they are posted, the clinical pharmacists must learn the additional clinical terms and abbreviations used in those wards. They should be able to convey their views and observations about the team clearly without mincing words. Thus, communication skills become an important prerequisite for ward rounds. Needless to point out, better communication is possible only when the person has a command over the language. English is the language that is usually used to communicate in a hospital among the health care team. However, the knowledge of the local language is also required to communicate with patients and their caretakers. Thus, at least a working knowledge in the local language has to be acquired wherever the clinical pharmacist is appointed.

While communicating with doctors and the other team members, the pharmacists should use polite, low pitch and firm words so as not to disturb the patients of the ward. Also, they must be careful while discussing side effects observed, alternate drugs suggested or doubt about drugs given so that they do not make the patient lose faith in the treatment. This might upset the patient. Similarly, they should make a wise choice of words so as not to hurt the feelings of the team members or their services. They must always remember that only faithful coordination among the team results in success.

Occasions may arise when the clinical pharmacists are required to give information or suggestion on a particular topic which they are not familiar with. They must honestly admit to the fact and assure the team to get the information when the ward round is completed. There is no need for bluffing or guessing the information. As promised, they must deliver the information as quickly as possible after the ward round.

Completion of Ward Round

Having discussed what to do before and during the ward round, let us move on to "what to do after the ward round". During the preparation for the ward round, the clinical pharmacists update the relevant documents. After the ward round is completed, they have to update these documents with additional information discussed and decided during the latest ward round. This information is noted briefly in a handheld case diary during ward rounds and elaborately written in the registers of the clinical pharmacy department.

Before attending to this work, the clinical pharmacists must give priority to the information that they are supposed to give to the team members. They may be urgently required by the team members to complete their records or to commence the follow-up treatment decided during the ward round. If no such work is there, they can attend to the updating work as discussed above. Thus, documentation is one of the major tasks after ward-rounds.

Moving on, the clinical pharmacists can communicate the decisions to other departments concerned, if relevant and necessary. They may have to communicate with hospital administration, the head of Nursing Services, the head of Pharmacy Services, the head of Lab

Services, and the head of dietary services. This information may be sent via e-mails, in writing or through phones. Acknowledgments can be collected through messengers and then filed.

Finally, clinical pharmacists have to communicate some of the decisions like change in therapy, drug or procedure to the patient or their caregivers. This has to be done carefully while counseling the patient. Thus, the patients are encouraged and their co-operation is ensured to continue the treatment. Sometimes, some parts of it or the entire work of this nature is assigned to the nurses also. In that case, the clinical pharmacist has to brief the nurse concerned about the matters related to clinical pharmacy services before such patient counseling sessions.

CONCLUSION

As discussed above, day-to-day, on the spot decisions are taken, depending on the disease manifestations, drug's effect, etc. This is done in the best possible way by the multidisciplinary team that ensures better treatment and achievement of its goal for which the entire team has put in its efforts. To chip in more contribution, clinical pharmacists should also specialize like medical professionals. After Pharm.D or M.Pharm pharmacy practice, clinical pharmacists can specialize in Pediatrics Pharmacy, Geriatric Pharmacy, Antibiotic therapy, Drug withdrawal treatment, Psychiatric pharmacy, etc, courses that are conducted in countries like the USA. If acquired, this qualification will take the clinical pharmacy services to a higher level and bring respect and glory to the profession of pharmacy.

MEDICATION HISTORY AND PHARMACEUTICAL CARE

INTRODUCTION

Pharmaceutical care is a new concept evolved during the middle of the 1970s after the pharmacists were given the responsibility of monitoring drug therapy in the 1960s. It is an extension of the clinical pharmacy services that started towards the end of the 1960s and developed into a full scheme of pharmaceutical care. Many functions assigned under this concept are new to pharmacists and hence, a section of them was reluctant to accept those responsibilities. These tasks involve monitoring, reviewing and documenting the therapy along with taking full responsibility for the result.

DEFINITION

Helper and Strand have defined, "Pharmaceutical care as the responsible provision of drug therapy for the purpose of achieving definite outcomes that improve a patient's quality of life"

FIP adopted the above definition with a little modification. They inserted the words 'or maintain' after the word 'improve' and thus, the new definition is,

"Pharmaceutical care is the responsible provision of drug therapy for the purpose of achieving definite outcomes that improve or maintain a patient's quality of life"

In certain disease conditions like AIDS or Diabetes, improving patient's quality of life is not always possible. Just maintaining it at the present level of quality, without further deterioration, itself is considered a significant achievement.

Pharmaceutical care and clinical pharmacy: The above definition looks similar to the definition of clinical pharmacy services. What is the difference between them? Roger Walker says, 'the practice of clinical pharmacy is an essential component in the delivery of pharmaceutical care.' He further elaborates, ' the delivery of pharmaceutical care is dependent on the practice of clinical pharmacy, but the key feature of care is that the practitioner takes responsibility for a patient's drug-related needs and is held responsible for that commitment. Thus "pharmaceutical care is a cooperative, patient-centered system for achieving specific and positive patient outcomes from the responsible provision of medicines" he concludes. From the above quote, it is clear that in pharmaceutical care, the pharmacist takes direct responsibility for the patient's drug-related needs and thereby, assures its quality in this care.

Types of Pharmaceutical care: As per the above definition, the pharmacist takes full responsibility for the drug therapy given to an individual patient under the concept of pharmaceutical care. Now, the question arises "who is responsible for the therapy given to the community as a whole under special circumstances"?. Here too, the pharmacists should provide pharmaceutical care. In this population-based pharmaceutical care, they have to use demographic or epidemiological data for serving the needs of society. According to a document published by WHO, it includes establishing hospital formulary, developing and networking pharmacy services, conducting and evaluating drug utilization review, developing and educating drug-related policies, etc. On the other hand, the first type of pharmaceutical care given to the individual patient involves monitoring drug therapy and modifying it, if necessary. Though pharmaceutical care is provided in cooperation with the entire health care team, a pharmacist alone is responsible for the cost, quality, and outcome of pharmaceutical care.

Basic Concept of Pharmaceutical Care

1. In pharmaceutical care, first, the pharmacist plans an individualized drug therapy for the patient. It aims at specific results and formulated in consultation with other health care professionals and patients.
2. For the above plan, the evidence is collected, its merits and demerits are studied and then adopted for implementation.
3. The patient is educated about the plan and its method of execution and
4. While the patient is under therapy, the outcomes are constantly monitored and modified, if required.

Thus, pharmacists in co-operation with other health care professionals and patients, design, implement and monitor a therapeutic plan that produces definite outcomes for the patient. These tasks are nicely presented by Helper et al in their paper "Opportunities and responsibilities in pharmaceutical care" published in 1990 in the American Journal of hospital pharmacy.

Pharmaceutical Care, for whom?

Though it is ideal to provide pharmaceutical care for all patients, in practice, it is not possible. Hence, patients should be selected on the basis of the following situations.

- Patients in critical conditions or diseases, that is, patients with cardiac problems, hypertension, diabetes, asthma, etc, should be given priority.

- Patients whose body conditions are vulnerable to adverse reactions, like patients with liver or kidney damage, pediatric and geriatric cases, etc

- Patients who are given risky drugs which are highly likely to cause damage, if wrongly used e.g. anticancer drugs, aminoglycosides, anticoagulants and

- Patients in acute conditions and when the drugs are given do not produce the desired level of therapeutic action, as in, certain infectious diseases and severe diarrhea.

When provided with pharmaceutical care, these risky patients can be saved with the co-operation and efforts of the entire health care team. Though pharmacists plan, execute and monitor the pharmaceutical care program, they have to ensure the support and active participation of the entire health care team to achieve the definite outcome planned.

Principle and Practice of Pharmaceutical Care

In 1995, the American Pharmacists Association [APhA] published 'the principles of practice for pharmaceutical care' to guide the concept of pharmaceutical care when it was started developing. In that document, it is pointed out what is needed to achieve the goal of pharmaceutical care and various steps involved in it. The following are the excerpts from the document:

To fulfill the objectives of pharmaceutical care,

- Pharmacists must establish a professional relationship with the patient and maintain it.

- Patient-specific medication information must be collected, organized, recorded and maintained

- The above information must be evaluated and a drug therapy plan developed mutually with the patient

- The pharmacist assures that the patient has all supplies, information, and knowledge necessary to carry out the drug therapy plan and

- The pharmacist reviews, monitors and modifies the therapeutic plan as necessary and appropriate in concert with the patient and health care team.

Steps Involved in the Practice of Pharmaceutical Care

1. **Medication history:** By medication history interview with the patient or with the patient's caretakers, old medical records, leftover medicines, etc, patient-specific data is collected first. This data must be complete and comprehensive in all aspects. All these data are recorded accurately and confidentially. It is shown to others only with the permission of the patient or if required by the law.

2. **Data Evaluation:** After evaluation, some decisions can be taken from the above data like the opportunity to improve the present condition, the effectiveness of planned therapy, way to reduce the future drug-related problem, etc. These decisions can be conveyed to the patient, to the extent necessary, in order to make them understand the present condition and future prospects.

3. **Designing a plan:** The pharmacists should design a plan to treat the patient with a specific achievable goal. For this, they can consult other health care professionals and enroll in their co-operation. After this, drugs suitable for the patient should be selected and then the ways of monitoring its effect have to be identified. The design can also include non-drug treatment, dietary changes, etc. It should also be clear about the therapeutic endpoint and monitoring limitations.

4. **Executing the plan:** The plan evolved as above should be implemented with care. During this stage, the pharmacist requires the support and involvement of other health care professionals, patient attendants and of course, the patient themselves. All the supplies starting from drug to other items should be ensured by the pharmacist in time.

5. **Monitoring the plan and outcome:** The pharmacist has to regularly monitor the outcome of the treatment to ensure satisfactory progress. If it is not up to the mark, the plan should be modified and then implemented. While monitoring the therapy, the patient's vital parameters should be checked using lab tests, whenever necessary. However, costly tests should be avoided as far as possible to keep the cost of treatment minimum and affordable to the patient as that is also one of the goals of pharmaceutical care. If positive outcomes are noticed, they should be conveyed to other health care professionals to elevate their confidence in the treatment plan. All these developments should be recorded in the patient's case diary or record so that the follow-up becomes easier. The patient's medical and pharmacy records should always be updated. Communications with other health care providers also should be recorded.

Requirements for Successful Pharmaceutical Care

American Pharmacists Association has listed the important requirements for the successful implementation of pharmaceutical care. They are,

1. Knowledge, skill and function of personnel
2. Systems for data collection, documentation and transfer of information
3. Efficient workflow processes
4. References, resources, and equipment
5. Communication skills and
6. Commitment to quality improvement and assessment procedures

If all these requirements are in place while implementing the program of pharmaceutical care, better results can be achieved to improve the quality of the patient's life.

Evaluation of Pharmaceutical Care Services

Any product or service provided to the society should be evaluated for its quality; pharmaceutical care is not an exemption. The quality of any service including health care services can be assured by evaluating its structure, process, and outcome, according to Donabedian. On completion of this evaluation, shortcomings can be rectified and thus, a better outcome for the patient can be achieved. The evaluation or quality assurance process starts with the focus on the patient, process and then the result. As described above, a patient-specific plan must be prepared and implemented with the cooperation of the team. The result obtained is evaluated in the light of set goals. The quality of pharmaceutical care can be assured if the resources or structure is properly mobilized and the plan is correctly executed.

DOSING PATTERN AND DRUG THERAPY BASED ON PHARMACOKINETIC AND DISEASE PATTERN

INTRODUCTION

The word pattern can be interpreted as design, orderly arrangement, regulation, etc. Thus, the dosing pattern can be the one in which a dosage regimen for a patient is designed or arranged in such a way to suit their condition. In patterns, we repeat something at a particular distance, time or space, hence, an orderly appearance for the overall scheme develops. Here, the treatment for a patient is designed in an orderly manner so as to derive maximum benefit for the patient with minimum trouble and cost to them.

Requirements for arriving at a Pattern

To arrive at a dosing pattern to treat a patient, we need to determine the following:

A]   Loading Dose

B]   Maintenance Dose

C]   Dosing route, method, and frequency

D]   Individualizing dose.

The correctness of the above parameters can be verified by Therapeutic drug monitoring [TDM]. Hence, a clinical pharmacist must undertake plasma drug concentration analysis whenever necessary and determine the drug, its dose, and frequency. Then, the drug has to be administered in an orderly manner. The dosing pattern thus determined goes a long way in achieving therapeutic efficacy and result. It has to be meticulously followed and it cannot be permanent since the patient's condition changes owing to certain factors. Hence, a new dosing pattern may be required during the course of the treatment.

A] LOADING DOSE: After the administration of the drug, its effect usually shows a characteristic temporal pattern. The effect starts after a small lag period and it increases to a maximum over a period of time and then decreases if the next dose is not administered. The drug's effect depends on its concentration in the blood which, in turn, varies due to pharmacokinetic factors like absorption, distribution, and elimination. Ultimately, the drug's effect relies on a concentration which is required to be effective. This concentration is known as Minimum Effective Concentration [MEC] and as long as it is available, the drug is still in effect in the body. If it goes below this level, the effect reduces and is not useful to the patient. Hence, for quick relief, this minimum concentration has to be reached as quickly as possible and maintained for a reasonable period of time. The dose required to achieve MEC is called a Loading Dose. It is also defined as the dose of a drug administered initially to bring the plasma concentration to a level anticipated during maintenance. It may be a single dose or a series of doses that are given at the beginning of the therapy. Alternatively, it can also be given as slow IV infusion over a period of time to avoid a sudden increase in drug concentration in sensitive patients. Usually, it is calculated by the following formula

Loading dose = Target Cp .Vss/F where,

Cp = Concentration of drug in plasma

Vss = Volume of Distribution at steady-state and

F = Fraction available for action [Bioavailability]

For example loading dose of Theophylline is calculated using Vd as follows:

Vd of Theophylline = 0.5L/Kg [approx]

Desired plasma concentration =10 mcg/ ml or 10 mg /L

But Vd =fD/Cp where f is bioavailability, D is the dose of drug administered and C is the plasma concentration desired

Since 'f' for Theophylline is 0.96 it is considered as 1

Thus, 0.5L/Kg =1D/10 mg /L

0.5 =D/10, Hence D =5mg /Kg or

350 mg for a 70 Kg patient.

The loading dose is usually large and given by injection or high oral dose. Hence, it may be dangerous if toxic effects occur due to the quick equilibrium of drugs with plasma. As a result of these considerations, thorough monitoring of the patients is essential as both lower and higher doses are problematic. The former has no use and the latter is harmful to the patient.

B] MAINTENANCE DOSE:

It is the dose essential to maintain the required concentration of the drug in plasma. This required concentration is the one that is targeted to achieve. It is otherwise known as targeted concentration and it has to be steadily available without variation and hence, this is also referred to as steady-state concentration. Once the targeted concentration is reached and in plasma for a reasonable time, the physician wants to maintain it steadily. Hence, the maintenance dose after the loading dose is administered to the patient which is determined by the following equation:

Maintenance dose = target Cp. CL/f where

CL = clearance and f = Bioavailability. It is obvious that to maintain a concentration inside the body the loss of it by way of clearance has to be compensated.

Dosing rate $=$ CL [clearance]

Drugs given via oral are subjected to first pass metabolic loss hence the above equation is modified to include the bioavailability

f. Dosing rate $=$ CL   .Css

Thus, the maintenance dose is equal to loss by clearance and subject to the bioavailability of the drug. The concept of loading dose and maintenance dose is useful for drugs with a short half-life. It is clear from the above discussion that bioavailability, the volume of distribution and clearance play an important role in determining the required steady-state plasma concentration. These parameters vary considerably between patients. Hence, plasma drug concentration should be measured and a revised dose rate should be calculated using the following formula if there is considerable variation in Cp

$$\text{Revised dose rate} = \frac{\text{Previous dose rate} \times \text{Target Cpss}}{\text{Measured Cpss}}$$

C] DOSING ROUTE, METHOD AND FREQUENCY:

While determining the maintenance dose, dosing route [e.g. Parenteral], dosing method [eg.IV, IM, SC] and dosing frequency [6 hourly,8 hourly] are determined. They are like warp and weft of a design weaved on a cloth to create the pattern. All the above factors influence the steady-state drug concentration. The following figures explain the effect of the dosing route, method, and frequency. The drug can be administered by continuous infusion, infrequent large doses, or by frequent small doses.

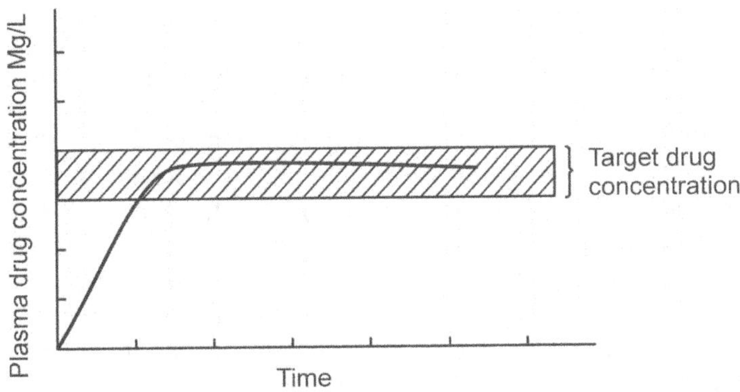

Fig. 17.2 Continues infusion of Drug (Falls within Therapeutic Range)

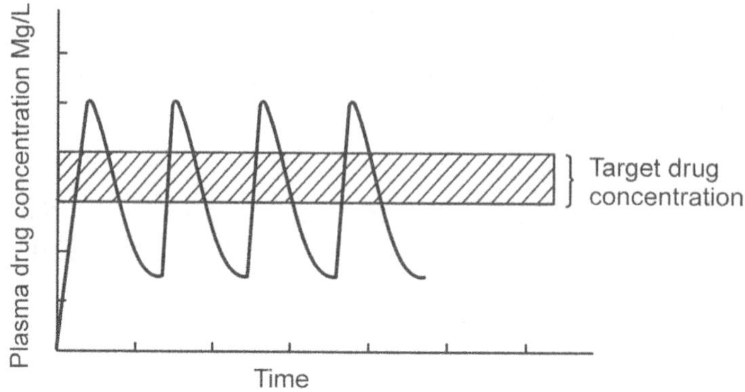

Fig. 17.3 Infrequent large Doses (Fluctuate above and below Therapeutic Range)

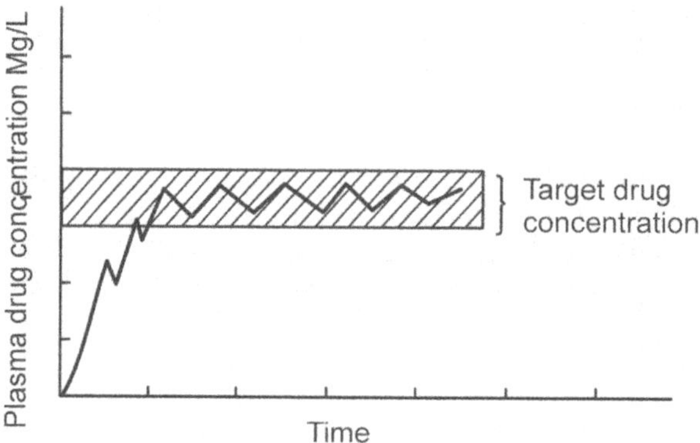

Fig. 17.4 Frequent small doses (remain within therapeutic range)

Figure 1 explains the continuous infusion, which is represented by a smooth curve that falls within the therapeutic range. Whereas, the infrequent large doses fluctuate above and below the target drug concentration, represented by peaks and troughs in Figure 2. On the other hand, frequent small dose method [Fig 3] results in a concentration within the therapeutic range and is more accepted and better suited to the patient as it involves the patient in taking their dose. However, many patients dislike frequent doses of drugs and their compliance with such a dosage regimen is questionable. This has to be taken into account while deciding the dosage pattern. But only when the patient sticks to the dosing pattern, the desired result can be expected. However, there is also a considerable and unpredictable amount of inter-patient variability in the pharmacokinetic parameters. Hence, individualizing the dose is required.

D] INDIVIDUALIZATION OF DOSE:

This is generally done based on pharmacokinetic parameters measured on an individual patient. It also depends on disease patterns. They are already discussed above.

QUESTIONS

1. Explain the need for individualization of dose briefly.
2. Write a short note on factors affecting bioavailability.
3. List the parameters useful in dose adjustment.
4. Write a note on preparation for a ward- round by pharmacist.
5. What are the skills needed for a ward round participation?
6. Explain the contribution of Clinical pharmacists in ward rounds.
7. Write a note on the principle and practice of Pharmaceutical care.
8. What are the requirements for successful Pharmaceutical care?
9. List the steps involved in the pharmaceutical care process
10. Write an essay about pharmacist's wards round participations
11. How will you individualize the dose for a patient?
12. Explain how pharmacokinetic parameters are interconnected?
13. Describe how the volume of distribution and clearance are calculated.
14. How and what affects the pharmacokinetic parameters? Why should a pharmacist intervene in those situations?
15. Define pharmaceutical care. How is it carried out? Explain.
16. Describe the concept of pharmaceutical care
17. Explain the requirements for arriving at a dosing pattern.

CHAPTER 18

OVER THE COUNTER (OTC) SALES

LEARNING OBJECTIVE

A useful topic in day to day community pharmacy practice is described in detail so that a community pharmacist can practice without rubbing the wrong side of the law enforcers or medical practitioners. A successful OTC sale practice ensure successful running of community pharmacy. On learning the chapter the reader can improve his skill as a pharmacist.

INTRODUCTION

Over the counter, [OTC] drugs are the medicines sold directly to a consumer over the counter without a prescription from a doctor. They are also called as non-prescription drugs. The OTC drugs are usually regulated by Active Pharmaceutical Ingredients present in it and not by the final product. Normally, they have ingredients that are safe and effective when used without a physician's care.

In India, OTC drugs are not yet defined by the government, and hence, it is assumed that any drug that does not fall into a prescription category is considered as an OTC drug. The lack of a legal definition for OTC drugs in India has led to this Rs 28,000 crore market segment being effectively unregulated.

REASONS FOR HUGE OTC MARKET

People often tend to purchase drugs from pharmacies without a prescription. There are many reasons for the same. 1. Due to prior exposure to symptoms of a disease, people consider they can purchase drugs once used by them again. 2. They often rely on the experiences gained by their close relatives and think they can use the same drug for similar conditions. 3. They take their present condition very lightly. 4. They are busy with their regular work and find little time to visit a doctor. 5. Many patients think purchasing OTC drugs would save doctor's fees, time, and transport cost 6. People also try to self diagnose and treat themselves based on the knowledge gathered from the internet and other sources. Thus, self-medication is growing day by day 7. Repeated, prolonged use of drugs, its popularity, and advertisement on TV and other media for OTC drugs lead to self-medication, resulting in OTC drug sales in large volumes.

COMMON CONDITIONS TREATED WITH OTC DRUGS

The following are the common conditions for which customers seek OTC drugs

- Headaches, Migraine, and fever   [Analgesics and Antipyretics]
- Upper respiratory tract infections, cough, cold and flu [Cough syrups, Lozenges, Gargles]
- Stomach pain, Heartburn and Acid reflux [Antacids]
- Muscle and Joint pain, Arthritis [NSAIDs]
- Allergies and Asthma [Bronchodilators]
- Small injuries, Wounds, and burns [Surgical dressings and ointments] and
- Athlete's foot, Corns and Acne [Topical preparations]

Advantages and Disadvantages of OTC Drugs

Advantages

- It ensures direct, rapid access to effective drugs.
- The easy and wide availability of drugs
- Decreased use of common healthcare system [Hospital resources]
- Allowing the individual to be in charge of their own health and
- Patients seeking drugs in the early stages of the disease [A responsible behavior]

Disadvantages

- Incorrect self-diagnosis, and hence, the OTC drugs become useless
- Increased risk of Drug-Drug interactions
- Increased risk of adverse events when not used appropriately
- Potential for misuse and abuse
- Delay in diagnosis of correct disease and consequently, increased complications

SALE OF OTC DRUGS

Owing to the reasons mentioned above, the OTC drug sale segment is the concern of all healthcare professionals, especially that of the pharmacists. The first concern of pharmacists is the patient's safety as people tend to purchase drugs for themselves as well as for their dependents. Since a pharmacist is not in a position to inquire with the patients who are away at home, they have to rely on the words of the purchaser. Hence, the safety of the patient becomes questionable and the pharmacist has to be extra careful when dispensing the OTC drugs. They should ensure there is a proper label on the container of the OTC drug and it is understandable by the patients. They should give the required advice and instructions regarding the OTC drug. While counseling the patient about the OTC drug, they should 1. Listen to the patient carefully 2. Question the patient thoroughly 3. Interpret their questions correctly and 4. Clear their doubts politely.

All these precautions are necessary to know the condition of the patients, their disease, its severity, and complications. If necessary, the pharmacist should guide the patient to a physician without dispensing the OTC drugs. To recall, all patients are considered as non-compliant as described in the chapter on non-adherence. Often, the pharmacist's instructions may not be followed faithfully. The misuse or abuse by way of forgetting the dose, doubling the dose, abrupt stopping of the drug are very common among patients. It is a very difficult task to promote the rational use of drugs among outpatients.

RATIONAL USE OF OTC DRUGS

It is very important to note that the irrational use of OTC drugs leads to complications in a patient. They may develop drug resistance or disease-causing organism could develop it further. Both conditions are dangerous to the patient and to society at large.

1. Ensure that there is no chance for drug-drug interaction. The OTC and prescription drugs may interact, if not prevented by the pharmacist. To avoid this, the patient must inform about the drugs they are already taking. Sometimes, the patients do not remember the name of the drug they are currently using and simply ignore the request of the pharmacist. Hence, general instruction to give a gap of an hour between the drugs should be conveyed.

2. There is a possibility of overdose for some drugs. Some ingredients may be present in more than one OTC drug, thereby overdose results. Hence, the patients should be enquired about the OTC drugs along with prescription drugs. For example, antihistamines, paracetamol, aspirin, and some decongestants may be present in many formulations for cold and nasal problems. If all these drugs are taken together, an overdose may be a possibility. Generally, healthcare professionals instruct the patient to stop all other drugs while taking the present drug.

3. Patients must be informed of the OTC drug's dose, contraindication, duration, and side effects

4. To avoid all these problems, the patients must be encouraged to purchase both prescription drugs and OTC drugs from the same pharmacy. Additionally, the pharmacist must pay attention to the drugs consumed, at least, by regular patients. Such a personalized service takes the pharmacist's respect among the customers to a much greater level and rational use of drugs by the patients can be ensured.

5. If the problem or disease persists or worsens, the patients should be instructed to stop OTC drugs and see a doctor.

6. Needless to mention, all drugs should be stored properly and kept out of reach of children.

MOVING PRESCRIPTION DRUGS TO OTC DRUGS LIST

Drugs standard control organization of all countries follows and watch the sale of the OTC drugs. Some greedy community pharmacies sell prescription drugs also along with the OTC drugs, ignoring the act and rules. Few prescription drugs are so effective, and hence, popular among the patients. The patients purchase them using old prescriptions or even without a prescription from the community pharmacists. Hence, drugs control departments of many governments move such drugs from prescription drug category to OTC drugs after considering the following factors:

1. **Long-time use of drugs:** If a drug is used for a long time, say 5 years and more, they can be moved to the OTC drugs list, subject to some conditions.

2. **High volume use:** Some drugs are so popular and have high acceptance by the patients. Hence, they are sold in high volumes and such drugs can be moved to the OTC category.

3. **No adverse report:** Long time use or high volume use alone cannot be the reason for declaring a drug as an OTC drug. There should not be any report of an adverse drug reaction or misuse of the drug during the above period.

4. Once a drug becomes popular, doctors stop prescribing them. Hence, it must be sold only through the OTC route, no other go, otherwise, manufacturers stop manufacturing them. This cannot be termed as a wise decision as people get deprived of their benefit. Denying them a popular and effective drug is unfair. Hence, the manufacturers apply to the department to move it to OTC drugs. A recent example is "Benadryl Expectorant", though it has a high dose of antihistamine, it is now promoted as OTC drug via an advertisement in TV and other media.

CONCLUSION

The sale of OTC drugs is like walking on the wall. There is always a danger of dispensing the wrong drug to the wrong patient. Also, there lies a temptation to sell prescription drugs along with OTC drugs. A pharmacist should control such temptations for their own welfare and that of patients. The OTC drug sales will be more than the prescription drugs sale in some pharmacies, especially those situated in a busy market area where the floating population is more. In fact, some pharmacies are thriving only with the sale of OTC drugs as prescription drug sales dried up after doctors started selling drugs (from the pharmacies attached to their clinics or hospitals). A pharmacy can be asked to adhere to the rules only when this practice is stopped as it is a question of survival for community pharmacies. The society will flourish only when all its members realize their responsibilities and function within their limits and not trespassing into each other's territories.

QUESTIONS

1. What are the common conditions treated with OTC drugs

2. List the advantages and disadvantages of OTC drugs

3. Write a note on the rational use of OTC drugs

Drug Store Management and Inventory Control

Learning Objective

The core of pharmacy practice is described in this chapter. Drug store management including its inventory control is the most useful topic and hence covered in detail. On complete understanding of the chapter the reader should be in a position to run his pharmacy in a successful manner. Almost all aspects of one of the important works of a pharmacist are explained here.

Introduction

"A store is a place for physical storage of materials that are carried around in a systematic manner in order to save them from any kind of damage, and exercising overall control on their movement". The act of organizing and managing a store is known as storekeeping.

Almost all organizations have one or more stores on their premises. For example, there are raw material stores, packing material stores, finished product stores for manufacturing companies, saleable goods for shops, at least, records and reports for the organizations not dealing with physical inventory. Thus, storekeeping should be known by all those involved in a healthcare organization including the pharmacists.

Importance of Store Keeping or Warehousing

Materials pilferage, deterioration, and careless handing lead to reduced profits or even major losses for an organization. It is more serious in the case of drugs and pharmaceuticals where improper storage practices lead to the loss in terms of money and human lives alike. Hence, the study of drugs storekeeping and management is very important for a pharmacist.

Types of Stores

There are 3 main types of stores:

1. Central stores where centralized buying and handling of drugs are undertaken.
2. Central stores with sub-stores: Here, buying is done at central stores but the handling is taken care of at various sub-stores and
3. Decentralized (or) Individual stores: Here, buying and handling of drugs are undertaken by the buyer and storekeeper of each department.

The type of stores adopted depends upon the circumstances prevailing in a hospital. The first two types of stores are common. In the first type (central stores), there are a few advantages:

1. The labor required for this storage is less compared to that of the decentralized storage.
2. The maintenance of the number of records is lower in this method.

However, the main disadvantage is that this store may not be under the control of a qualified person. By appointing a couple of assistant storekeepers with relevant qualifications, we can solve this problem to a great extent.

In the decentralized method of storage, the main advantage is that it is under the control of a qualified person (pharmacist). They can adjust the inventory based on the prescribing trends and that is another advantage of this method of storage.

Organization of Drug Store

In order to organize a drug store in a hospital, the following points should be considered:

(a) Location and layout

(b) Design of store building

(c) Management

(a) **Location and layout:** The normal practice is to locate the drug store near the consuming department, that is, near the outpatient dispensary and wards. The important points to keep in mind regarding the location of stores are:

- Easy movement of materials.
- Good housekeeping.
- Sufficient space for men and material handling.
- Optimum use of storage space like the floor, racks, shelves, etc.
- Proper preservation from rain, sunlight, and animals.
- The volume and variety of goods to be handled and
- Accessibility to the mode of transportation such as lorry, van, etc.

(b) **Design of stores building:**

(i) **Building:** The stores building must have adequate facilities for the preservation of drugs. Facilities such as cold storages, air conditioning, and similar facilities should be provided.

The building must be strong, spacious, high enough, well-ventilated, and neatly arranged. The floor must be strong to withstand the pressure of frequent movement of materials.

(ii) Lighting: The lighting must be clear and adequate and at the same time, windows should be kept open to a minimum. There must be proper generator facilities in case of power failure, both for lighting and cold storage facilities.

(iii) Safety: The ways inside the stores must be kept clean, free from obstructions. This is to make sure that the movement inside the stores is not affected or results in accidents. The provision of fire fighting facilities is necessary for important places, especially where inflammable materials like chloroform, ether, etc., are stored and handled. The entry of unauthorized staff and persons should be strictly prohibited and the drug store should be kept under proper lock, wherever necessary.

(c) Management: See below

Types of Materials Stored

1. Tablets
2. Capsules
3. Injections
4. Ointments, pastes, and creams
5. Liquid orals, and
6. Chemicals

If not stored separately in a surgical store of the hospital, the following materials are also stored in the medical/drug store of the hospital under the control of a pharmacist.

- Bed sheets/blankets
- Bedside tables
- Cot
- LVP stands (saline stands)
- Needles
- Medical Gases
- Syringes
- Surgical gloves
- Surgical dressings like bandages, gauze, cotton, etc.
- Surgical equipment and instruments like scissors, forceps, etc.
- Surgical suture and ligatures
- Trolleys
- Wheelchairs etc.

Store Room Arrangement

The storeroom can be arranged by various methods like alphabetically, pharmacologically, supplier wise, formulation wise, etc. Each of these methods has its own advantages and disadvantages. Usually, in a big store like a hospital store, formulation wise arrangement is followed. Thus, the drugs are arranged, as follows:

1. Capsules
2. Chemicals
3. External use preparations
4. Injections
5. Liquid orals and
6. Tablets

Each one of these formulations is arranged alphabetically within their respective areas of storage for easy location and issue. Moreover, there should always be adequate extra space for shelves in each of these areas for future requirements. Thus, keeping one type of formulation, say tablets, in different places of the store can be avoided.

Category Wise Storage of Inventory

There are many ways of exercising control over the inventory. For example, drugs can be stored according to their cost, supply source or utility. As mentioned above, each method of storage has its merits and demerits, and hence, the storekeeper has to decide which method is more convenient for them and the organization. As the inventory is analyzed for cost, source or utility, methods are referred to as ABC analysis, GOLF analysis, and VED analysis.

ABC analysis: Here the drugs are grouped according to the cost of the material as shown below:

'A' group items: This includes costly items such as biologicals and antibiotics. These items may not contribute to 10% of the total inventory, but they consume over 70% of the total inventory cost.

'B' group items: These items are neither costly nor cheap. They usually represent 20% of the total inventory and the total investment on these items also does not exceed 20%.

'C' group items: These items are less expensive items but occupy 70% of the total stock and the total cost does not exceed 10%.

Disadvantages of ABC analysis: The critical and the most essential items for production or distribution may be included in the C category on account of not being too costly or too cheap. For example, magnesium stearate or talc in the manufacture of tablets, needles or plasters in case of surgical items, water for injections in case of drugs are cheaper compared to other items in these categories. But if they are not available for any reason, there may be a huge problem in the manufacture, surgery or treatment respectively.

GOLF analysis: Here, the drugs are grouped on the basis of the source of supply of the drug. Thus,

G -   Government controlled items

O -   Open market items

L -   Local purchase items and

F -   Foreign items are stored according to this order

This is an arbitrary method of classifying drugs. It may not always be possible for a storekeeper to classify drugs according to this category. Hence, it is not followed often.

VED analysis: Here, the drugs are classified on the basis of their utility.

where,   V-   Vital items

      E -   Essential items and D -   Desirable items

Vital items like life-saving drugs are very important without which a hospital cannot function. Essential items are a little less important as compared to the vital items. However, they are always available. Desirable items are not important compared to the first two categories. Their unavailability does not cause any major problems. Some stores are arranged according to this method.

Storage of Drugs

Management of a Drug Store

1. **Manpower:** To manage a drug store, the first requirement is manpower. Thus, in order to organize drug stores in a hospital, qualified staff (pharmacists) must be appointed in adequate numbers to manage the store. In addition to pharmacists, a sufficient number of clerical staff and laborers should be appointed to maintain accounts and to physically handle the materials respectively.

2. **Orderly arrangement:** As mentioned earlier, drugs can be arranged on the shelves either alphabetically, pharmacologically or formulations wise like capsules, tablets, and injections, etc. Regardless of the method, the drugs should be easily traceable for instant issuing.

The costly items must be kept locked similar to narcotic drugs. The heavy materials must be stored near the entrance or exit for obvious reasons. Vaccines, sera, suppositories, and similar substances which require cold storage should be stored in refrigerators.

Markings on the Inventory

In order to locate, identify and know a few details about a particular item, some markings are made either on the product or on the place of storage. There are floor marking, shelf stripping, and goods markings for the above purposes.

Floor markings: In the wooden or concrete floor of the stores, the name of the item stored in the particular area is marked by paint.

Shelf stripping: Paper, card, plastic, or metallic strips are used for shelf stripping in which the name of the item is written. Thus, the name of the item is clearly visible and it is easier to locate them.

The advantages of these types of markings are:

1. A particular area is allotted for a particular product
2. It brings orderliness
3. Checking the stock becomes easier

Goods marking: In this method, the date of receipt of goods, cost price, and supplier names are marked near or on the goods. The cost price is marked in code words. So, it is easy to determine the discount while selling. Similarly, if different suppliers exist for a single product, goods marking helps in easy identification of the source of supply.

Card system: All the stored items are entered in separate cards with name, manufacturer, supplier, invoice no. and date, batch number, quantity, expiry date, and other details needed to refer to the particular item. The receipt and issues are entered on the card right there to update the information about that item. This card must be kept close to the item. Now that the inventory is computerized, this may be an outdated method of inventory control. However, a lot of hospitals are still following this system, sometimes as a measure to double-check.

Stock checking: The hospital can assign the duty of physically checking the stock of drugs to certain people and they should perform their duty with or without notice to the employees of stores. The closing balance on the stock card must tally with actual balance. The damaged or expired drugs should be disposed of after necessary sanctions from the authorities.

Records: Every store should maintain the record for its purchase, issue, and stock of drugs. All these entries in their register should have supportive documents like invoices, indents, and other important documents. They should be maintained up to the date.

Thus, a store should be managed by the pharmacist in a professional and efficient manner. The efficiency of drug store management reflects on the following aspects:

1. It must be able to purchase quality drugs at a minimum cost.
2. It should systematically store, maintain, and preserve the drugs.
3. There should be no interruption in the drug supply.
4. The suppliers should be promptly paid with no complaints from them like delayed payment or part payment etc.
5. All facilities to prevent theft, pilferage, damage, and fire accidents must be available and
6. Physical verification of stocks for expiry dates and stability must be undertaken as often as possible.

Storage Conditions

Storage conditions stipulated in each product must be followed in order to maintain its safety and potency. Hence, a store pharmacist must be thorough with the storage conditions of drugs. General guidelines like 'protect from sunlight', 'protect from moisture' etc. should be strictly followed. Some products may be required to be stored in certain conditions under a specific temperature. Storing at either sides of the temperature leads to unwanted problems. The conditions of storage, even though given in general terms, are defined in all pharmacopeias including the Indian pharmacopeia. They are:

(a)   **Cold:** Any temperature not exceeding $8°C$ and usually between $2°C$ to $8°C$

(b)   **Cool:** Any temperature between $8°C$ to $25°C$

(c)   **Room temperature:** The temperature prevailing in a working area ($25°C$ to $30°C$)

(d)   **Warm:** Any temperature between $30°C$ to $40°C$

(e)   **Excessive heat:** Any temperature above $40°C$

(f)   **Protect from freezing:** Freezing results in loss of strength or change in the characters of the drug, in addition to the risk of breaking the container. Hence, it must be carefully followed.

(g)   If no specific condition is given, it is understood as protection from light, moisture, freezing, and excessive heat.

PURCHASE AND INVENTORY CONTROL

INTRODUCTION

Purchase and inventory control are very important operations of a hospital pharmacy. Both of these tasks vary with the size of the hospital, distance from the source of supply, storage facilities, turn over, and cost. Usually, in a hospital, the HOD of hospital pharmacy or the Chief Pharmacist and a few other senior pharmacists are assigned these tasks. They have the expertise, experience, and endurance to carry out and complete them successfully. However, a budding pharmacist is expected to know the theoretical aspects of it and may be required to apply it in practice or even assist the seniors sometimes. The knowledge of purchase and inventory control is required even if the pharmacists decide to open their own community pharmacy store.

DEFINITIONS

As the three words, 'purchase' 'inventory' and 'control' are to be used repeatedly in this chapter, it is better to define them first. According to W.E. Hassan,

'Purchase' is defined as an act of getting something by paying money or its equivalent or simply to obtain or buy something for a price.

'Inventory' is defined as an itemized list of goods with their estimated worth, especially an annual account of stock taken in any business.

'Control' is defined as an act of exercising power over something.

Purchase or Procurement

Purchasing authorities: Once we decide to purchase something for an organization, the first question asked is, who should purchase or who has the authority to purchase. Then only, other aspects like what, where, when and how to purchase arise.

There are two views on the authority to be designated for purchasing. One view is all institutional purchases should be centralized and a purchase officer should be appointed for the purpose. Another view is that drugs and other related items are specialty items that require technical skills, and hence, the purchase should be assigned to a pharmacist. However, it all varies with the policies of the government or management of the hospitals. For example, there is only one centralized agent at the state level for the purchase of drugs and other items for all the hospitals in the state of Tamilnadu (Tamilnadu Medical Services Corporation, Chennai). Some other governments have a similar arrangement as it has many advantages like better control of inventory, bulk purchase, consequent large discounts, and prevention of malpractices and corruption at various levels.

However, if there are purchases at the institutional level and a purchase officer is appointed for the purpose, they are expected to work in collaboration with the Chief Pharmacist or HOD of the pharmacy services, each recognizing the importance of the function of the other. In this system, the pharmacist provides the specifications for the drugs to be purchased and has the authority to reject any article which may be below the standard and specifications. So, there may be either one of the above authorities available for purchasing drugs for a hospital.

(a)   In small hospitals, the purchasing function may be looked after by the officer in charge of stores or the hospital superintendent with the help of the storekeeper. As these officers have this work as an additional duty and they perform it along with their regular duties, they minimize the work and heavily depend on the storekeeper who may be a pharmacist.

The following are the **functions of purchasing authority** whether they are a purchase officer or a pharmacist. First of all, they must collect the purchase request form called an indent from the pharmacy. After its approval by higher authorities, the purchase order should be issued to the suppliers. All the records and documents pertaining to purchase should be properly maintained so that the follow-up actions in case of delayed supply or discrepancy in supply can be verified in the future. In order to get drugs at an economical price, competitive bidding must be arranged by those who are responsible for the purchase. Similarly, quotations for the required items can be obtained from various suppliers by sending the list of requirements with specifications.

(b)   The role of the pharmacists is very limited in purchasing drugs in the Indian hospitals as we employ only D. Pharm holders as pharmacists who are easily dominated. A complete department of pharmacy services with graduate and post-graduate pharmacists is yet to be established in our hospitals. However, pharmacists are supposed to know their future roles in drug procurement. There are some pre-requisite before purchasing drugs for the hospital. The role of a pharmacist begins with the preparation of the list of manufacturers, wholesalers or their local representatives with their addresses and phone numbers. They should keep the specifications for the drugs to be purchased ready. Then only they can prepare the purchase request form or indent and send it to the purchasing authority. After the approval, drugs can be purchased from various sources depending on quantity and management's policy. The following are the suppliers of drugs to hospitals.

1. Manufacturers of drugs

2. Wholesalers

3. Retailers (in case of emergency)

4. Tender winners and

5. Contract suppliers

The pharmacist is required to inform about these sources to the purchase officer and the choice of supplier is either made by the pharmacist or left to the discretion of the purchase officer. Irrespective of the way of purchasing, the pharmacist and authorities should make arrangements for testing the quality and standards of the drugs supplied to the hospital. It can be tested in the hospital's own testing lab, if available; otherwise, the samples can be sent to the commercial testing laboratories or government laboratories. The order for purchase is later executed, depending on the analytical report of the samples received. After receiving the goods, the pharmacist should acknowledge it in a proper format. If any item is to be returned to the supplier for any reason, they should prepare and submit a return goods memo and send it to the purchasing authority. The same procedure can be repeated after all the drugs are supplied and tested randomly for quality and then the payment for the same is recommended to the hospital management.

In order to perform the above duties, especially for preparing specifications, the pharmacists should refer to standard books like IP, BP, USP, National formulary, Pharmaceutical Codex, etc.

Purchase Procedure

The initiation for purchase of drugs starts from the pharmacists. After determining the drugs, their specifications, price, required quantity, etc., the pharmacist should prepare a purchase request form. This form has all the details mentioned above in addition to the available balance, anticipated monthly use, etc. The original copy of this form is sent to the administrative officer in charge of the department and upon the approval, it is forwarded to the purchasing department. A duplicate copy is maintained in the pharmacy department.

On receiving the purchase request form, the purchase officer prepares purchase orders in multiple copies which contain all the specifications, quantity, and other details that are taken from the request form. The first copy of the purchase order is sent to the manufacturers, suppliers or their representatives. The second copy is accounts payable and is sent to the accounts department and kept in the file until the goods are supplied and the received report comes from the initiating department. The third copy is retained by the purchase officers themselves for records and follow-up. The fourth one is sent to the initiating department i.e., the pharmacy. Upon receiving this copy, the pharmacist should compare it with the purchase request form for accuracy and modifications.

The fifth and the sixth copies are sent to the goods receiving department for verification and the received report is sent to the accounts department in the fifth copy. If the goods are to be ordered again, the sixth copy can be used or ignored.

If some goods are returned to the supplier for some reason, a return goods memo is prepared in multiple copies and sent to the initiating department, purchase officer, accounts department, and the stores.

Immediately after the goods are received, they are promptly entered in the purchase record and the stock register with all the relevant details, like, invoice number and date, name of the supplier, quantity received, etc.

Whenever an item is not supplied and is out of stock in the pharmacy and stores, an out of stock form should be prepared in duplicate and sent to the initiating or the consuming department so that a false sense of heavy demand is not created.

Control on Purchases

Almost all the superior authorities or management of the hospitals attempt to limit the purchase volume by placing an upper limit in rupees terms on the purchase order. This method may not serve the purpose, as it is easily circumvented by issuing multiple small orders or results in fewer items and quantities, causing, shortage of drugs in the hospitals.

A more scientific method of control on purchases is to calculate the inventory turnover and order the goods accordingly. It is calculated by dividing the cost of goods sold or issued during the financial year by the average of opening and closing inventory costs. This gives the number of times the inventory has been turned over during the period.

For example, if the total cost of goods sold or issued in one year in a big hospital is Rs. 20 Lakhs, the opening inventory cost is Rs. 6 Lakhs, and the closing inventory cost is Rs. 4 Lakhs, then the average of it is calculated to be Rs. 5 Lakhs. On dividing the total cost of Rs. 20 Lakhs by this average gives a turnover rate of 4.

Inventory turnover of 4 times a year indicates that the purchase was carried out properly in the previous year. That is, the goods are purchased on an average of once in 3 months and it is considered as a satisfactory practice in the trade. This turnover rate can be up to 6, meaning a purchase of goods once in 2 months, if the organization is running short of finance. But if it is more than 6, it denotes a pessimistic attitude of management and losing bulk purchase discounts. The pharmaceutical manufacturers offer more incentives on bulk purchases. For example, if you purchase 10 bottles of cough syrup, they give 1 bottle free. At the same time, if you purchase 25 bottles, 3 bottles are given for free. Similarly for 50, ten bottles and for 100 twenty-five bottles are offered, thus, decreasing your cost of purchase by 10% to 25% [or increasing your profit margin from 10% to 25%]. Moreover, repeated purchases of the same item multiple times in a year involve the cost of purchase every time and the waste of time and energy in the process of purchasing.

On the other hand, a low turnover rate [less than 4] indicates duplication of stock, large purchases of slow-moving items and dead stock and investment.

Thus, the purchases should be controlled in an efficient and reasonable manner. In order to do that, the purchasing authorities must know important aspects of inventory control. They are discussed below:

Inventory Control

While inventory is defined as an itemized list of goods with their estimated worth or value, inventory control is defined as a process of safeguarding the company's inventory and maintaining it at an optimum level.

The importance and uses of inventory control are listed below:

1. It reduces the cost of production
2. It minimizes the time wastage due to a shortage of raw materials
3. It minimizes the wastage of goods
4. It minimizes the capital investment
5. It maximizes customer service
6. It helps to deliver the goods at the right place and right time.
7. The value of goods on storage can be seen at any time and
8. It improves the overall handling and storing of goods.

Inventory Levels

While stocking goods, the inventory level should be optimum. Excess of stock leads to a huge cost of running the organization. At the same time, less stock leads to several problems in the supply of required items at the required time. Hence, storekeepers follow some levels of stock and they are,

1. **Maximum level:** A level is fixed after studying various factors, beyond which the materials should not be purchased at any time. This level is called maximum level.
2. **Minimum level:** It is a level beyond which the materials should not be allowed to fall at any time.
3. **Re-order level:** This is the level at which the order should be placed to replenish the stock.

Methods

Following are the various method of inventory control:

1. **Periodic inventory control:** In this method, a physical count of inventory at the end of each accounting period (a year) is undertaken.
2. **Perpetual inventory control:** In this method, entries are made in the register when the sale or issue is completed. Day-to-day entries thus made keep the record updated. This is the method of inventory control followed in all the dispensaries and medical stores of the hospital as an item or medicine going out of stock without knowing will create a lot of problems for the hospital.

3. **Special inventory -Inventory for perishable drugs:** Important life-saving drugs like biologicals, (antibiotics vaccine, serum, etc.,) which undergo degradation easily and have short shelf-life should be in special care. This can be achieved by the following methods:

(a)   Maintaining separate records for these items with their names, potencies and expiry dates.

(b)   Replacing the items nearing expiry or expired with the new ones by constantly checking the record as well as the physical stock.

Control of Inventory

Hospital pharmacists must control the inventory by using various measures available for the purpose. They are EOQ (Economic Order Quantity) and RQL (Re-order Quantity Level). These measures can also be used to control the purchase volume.

RQL: The greatest dilemma for a pharmacist during their professional practice in a medical store (of a hospital or outside) is when and how much of an item of medicine is to be ordered. An arbitrary decision on these aspects will definitely lead to trouble and loss. Hence, a scientific method is needed, based on which a rational decision can be made by the pharmacist.

One of the methods to determine the time of order placing is RQL (Re-order Quantity Level). It is the level that must be reached before additional stocks are ordered. Sapp, et al., has developed a table to use EOQ and RQL. According to this, for determining the re-order quantity, the average usage rate per month in units of the issue should be divided by 13 weeks. The number is then multiplied by the average Vendor Lead Time (VLT) plus the safety factor. The following table illustrates the point:

VLT	Safety factor
0 to 2 weeks	1.0
2 to 5 weeks	1.5
5 to 8 weeks	2.0
8 to 11 weeks	2.5
11 to 15 weeks	3.0

$$RQ = \frac{\text{Average usage rate per month}}{13} = A$$

$$= A \times (VLT + SF)$$

A simpler method of getting RQL is by multiplying lead time in days by average daily usage of the inventory. For example, if you are dispensing on an average 20 bottles of B.Complex syrup per day and it requires 7 days for the supplier to deliver the goods, then you must order when your stock reaches 140 [20 × 7] bottles.

EOQ (Economic Order Quantity): The quantity of the item is to be ordered is determined by using the EOQ factor. To calculate this factor, it is important to ascertain the cost of ordering and the cost of carrying the inventory or holding cost. Then the EOQ is calculated by applying the following formula:

$$EOQ = \frac{2 \times 12 \times \sqrt{\text{monthly usage} \times \text{cost of ordering}}}{\text{Unit cost} \times \text{Holding cost}}$$

It may be advantageous to order expensive items on a monthly basis and inexpensive items annually. Another method of calculating the EOQ is by mathematical approach. Here the formula used is,

$$EOQ = \sqrt{\frac{2AB}{C}}$$

Where,

A is Annual usage of inventory in units

B is Buying cost per order

C is Carrying cost per unit

Example: If A = 1600 units, B = 50 Rs and C = 1Re, then

$$EOQ = \sqrt{\frac{2 \times 1600 \times 50}{1}} = 400 \text{units}$$

However, in this method there are some limitations, they are,

1. The sale per year is an assumption.
2. Time taken for supply is not considered.
3. If there is unexpected demand, this calculation is useless and
4. The EOQ calculated as above may be in fraction.

Nevertheless, instead of arbitrarily determining these quantities without any criteria, it is better to use some scientific calculations. A pharmacist will learn these and other skills with the experience in the job. Majority of the times, calculations made using discretion and experience of a pharmacist will be correct and rewarding.

QUESTIONS

1. List the types of stores
2. What is an ABC analysis?
3. What is GOLF analysis?
4. What is VED analysis?
5. Write a note on marking on the inventory
6. What is inventory control?
7. What are the different inventory levels?
8. What are the different methods of inventory control?

9. What is the inventory turnover rate? How it is calculated?

10. What is RQL?

11. What is EOQ?

12. How is a drug store organized?

13. How is a drug store managed?

14. Explain the category wise storage of inventory. Discuss its advantages and disadvantages.

15. Write in detail about the storage of drugs. Add a note on storage conditions of drugs.

16. Explain the drug purchase procedure of a Hospital. Enumerate the role of pharmacists in it.

17. How is the inventory controlled in a hospital? Explain various methods and calculations involved.

18. How is the purchase controlled in a hospital or in a medical store? Discuss the effect of excess or fewer purchase quantities.

19. Enumerate the role of purchasing authorities in the purchase of drugs for a hospital?

CHAPTER 20

INVESTIGATIONAL USE OF DRUGS

LEARNING OBJECTIVE

The chapter's objectives are to give an elaborate account of the investigational use of drugs. Thus it deals with principles, guideline, classification, control and identification of investigational drugs. By specifying the role of pharmacist and advisory committee formed for the purpose, it focuses on almost all aspect of the topic. The student should able to adopt it while in practice.

INTRODUCTION

'An investigational drug is a substance that has been tested in the laboratory and approved by the drug control department for testing on people. Such drugs that are approved for one disease or condition still considered as investigational drugs if they are used for another disease.'

PRINCIPLES INVOLVED

There are certain principles for undertaking the investigation of a new drug. The first and foremost principle to be followed is informed consent from the people volunteering for testing the drugs. The second important principle is safety, that is, the drug that is used should be safe for the patient and the staff. Additionally, it should not jeopardize the safety of the institution where the testing is done. The third principle is to follow ethical, legal, and scientific standards. Let us study these principles in detail.

1. **INFORMED CONSENT:** It is the consent from the patient or person [volunteer] on whom the drug is to be tested after being fully informed about the risks involved in the study. It is the duty of the investigators to explain all aspects of the study in a manner that is understandable. There should be no hidden or partially explained facts. If the risks involved are not known, that should also be informed to the patient. For this, the patient should be of sound mind and matured enough to understand the briefing. If the patient is in an advanced

stage of the disease and the new drug is going to be used as a last resort to save him, the above details should be explained to the patient's guardian or caretaker. The consent should be obtained from the patient or volunteer in writing in the specific format available for the purpose. The patient should also be informed that they have every right to withdraw from the study at any time during the course of the investigation. It is all the more important to obtain consent without using any force, fraud or influence. The problem with this aspect of the investigation is that it is easier to deceit people in our country with a pool of uneducated people.

2. **SAFETY:** The second important principle is the safety of the people involved in the investigation. The new drug under investigation may be a hazardous chemical, an antigen like microorganism, herbal formulation with unknown active constituents, or chemicals formed after formulation. Hence, the investigating team should be careful and vigilant from the beginning of the study regarding the safety of everyone involved. Since the investigational drug is to be administered to the patient, their safety acquires topmost priority and thorough monitoring on a regular basis. The investigators that are directly involved in the study should also take all the precautionary self-safety measures and strictly adhere to the rules and follow good laboratory practices [GLP]. The safety of the institution is also important as the treatment of patients with infectious diseases, potent microorganisms, inflammable or hazardous chemicals, all pose a great danger to the institution and even to the surrounding environment.

3. **STANDARDS:** There are a few important standards to be followed while undertaking the investigation of new drugs. These are legal, ethical, and scientific standards. The ethical standard is the one which should be followed as per the direction of the national and institutional ethical committee. In fact, only after obtaining an undertaking from the investigator permission is given. The ethical committee has the moral responsibility to monitor the study. Similarly, the investigation must follow the law of the land where the study is being conducted. In this case, the law enforcing authority is the drug control department and they should conduct periodical inspections including surprise visits to make sure the investigation is not violating any law of the country. The next standard to be adhered to is the scientific standard where the investigating team is expected to follow the established scientific methods of investigation. Even when a new procedure is to be followed, it should be validated by the authorities including the ethical committee. There should be no room for compromises in following the scientific standards citing lack of procedure, equipment, chemicals, drugs or expert of the field.

CLASSIFICATION: Investigational drugs can be classified either by their position in the research scheme or the nature of the investigation itself. In the first type of classification, a research drug may be in the preliminary stage of investigation or after the completion of the study. In the second type of classification, the investigation itself can be for commercial or research purposes. Either way, the classification revolves around the investigational new drug [IND]

An application for IND is submitted after the completion of thorough animal studies that establish that the proposed drug is reasonably safe to use in humans and it has the potential to market as a drug for treatment. Thereby, its commercial development is justified. Some drugs, which are either new or already in the market can also be investigated to find out new indications, methods of treatment or dosage forms. Thus, they form the part of the second classification (research purpose).

Usually, after the completion of the preliminary stage of an investigation, the dosage form studied can be [Tablet, Capsule, Liquid Oral or External use preparation] manufactured in a small quantity and given to select dispensaries for dispensing to a select group of patients. It can also be dispensed to a larger population on prescription by the principal investigator or co-investigators. Thus, the position of an investigational new drug in the research pipeline varies with the progress of the research and classified accordingly.

CONTROL: The investigational use of drugs is controlled by various authorities at its various stages of research. Nowadays, clinical research organizations [CRO] are established purely for the purpose of clinical trials of the drugs. They have their own hospital to carry out small scale studies. Sometimes, they have a tie-up with big hospitals for large scale studies involving hundreds of patients. In that case, the principal investigator of the CRO or the investigator employed in the same hospital should provide full information about the drug to the PTC of the hospital. They are 1. New drug number, 2.Generic name, 3.Chemical name 4. Proprietary name, if any, 5.Manufacturer detail, 6.General chemistry, 7.Pharmacology, 8.Toxicology, dose range, Method and route of administration, 9.Antidote [if known] and 10. Therapeutic uses.

This information is passed on to doctors, nurses and pharmacists of the hospital either in full or required parts. A couple of members of the investigating team remain with the patients round the clock to monitor the outcome of the treatment. The hospital team and the investigation team should coordinate properly.

IDENTIFICATION OF INVESTIGATIONAL DRUG

Usually, the hospitals follow the practice of affixing a different label for investigational drugs for easy identification. Some hospitals print the label in red color to draw the attention of the health care team. Sometimes, special labels are prepared with the patient's name, doctor's name, and research drug number, etc. so as to follow the investigation without a mix-up. It is one of the major tasks of the pharmacist, co-opted in the research team. Other roles of the pharmacists are discussed below:

ROLE OF HOSPITAL PHARMACIST

If an ideal hospital pharmacy, full with manufacturing facilities is available in a hospital, there are few valuable roles that a hospital pharmacist can play in the research. For example, they can prepare placebo drugs in the exact same dosage form as that of the investigational drug. Needless to point out, the placebo plays a crucial role in the study of treatment outcomes. Similarly, the pharmacist can prepare a new dosage form of the investigation drug, if the permission is obtained earlier by including it in the original application. Thus, a tablet can be substituted with a capsule or liquid oral. The tablet can also be enteric-coated or sugar-coated or made a sustained release. These dosage forms help in the pharmacokinetic studies due to their varied bioavailability, excretion, etc.

Thus, the clinical pharmacist in the team will perform therapeutic drug monitoring [TDM] by carrying out pharmacokinetic studies in full. The variations in absorption, distribution, metabolism, and excretion [ADME] of the drug can be detected and informed to the investigator. This valuable contribution of the clinical pharmacist will be appreciated by the research team. Thus, not only the drug manufacturing pharmacist but also the analytical and clinical pharmacists become an integral part of the investigational use of drugs and clinical trials.

ADVISORY COMMITTEE

As the investigational use of new drugs is in practice for a long time in the USA, they have perfected the process. They have the bucca Advisory committee for this purpose. Their constitution, function, and experiences are mentioned on the USFDA website. The Indian pharmacists can benefit to a great extent by emulating USFDA example. Hence, it is quoted below extensively with due acknowledgment and gratitude.

"The Food and Drug Administration of USA regulates more than 150,000 marketed drugs and medical devices. At any time, nearly 3,000 investigational new drugs are being developed. More dietary supplements than ever before are on the market, and Americans today have a much broader range of food choices. Then, there are the scores of blood products and veterinary medicines for which the FDA is responsible".

Access to this growing range of products offers opportunities for advancing public health and improving people's lives. But it also creates new vulnerabilities and greater potential risks for people who use the products. To keep up with the challenges that the FDA's full-time experts face when reviewing innovative and rapidly evolving technologies, the agency hires "special government employees" whose opinions complement its goals to provide safe and effective products.

These third-party advisors make up the FDA's technical and scientific advisory committees. The primary role of an advisory committee is to provide independent advice that will contribute to the quality of the agency's regulatory, decision-making and lend credibility to the product review process. In this way, the FDA can make sound decisions about new medical products and other public health issues. And although the advisory committees have a prominent role in the product approval stage, they are sometimes included earlier in the product development cycle and are asked to consider issues relating to products already in the market.

The Committees are typically asked to comment on the adequate data support approval, clearance, or licensing of a medical product for marketing. The advisory committees also may recommend the FDA's request for additional studies and suggest changes to a product's labeling. However, their recommendations should not bind the agency to any decision. While committee discussions and final votes are very important to the FDA, the final regulatory decision rests with the agency.

The advisory committee meetings often receive a considerable amount of media attention, and the agency welcomes such scrutiny because it helps provide public assurance of a responsible process.

Committee Members and Participants

The rapidly expanding technology in food and drugs in the 1960s led to a growing opinion among scientists and other public health experts that the FDA could perform its mission of consumer protection more effectively by using public advisory committees. With the passage of the Federal Advisory Committee Act in 1972, Congress prescribed the formal use of advisory committees throughout the federal government.

According to the law, membership in advisory committees must be "fairly balanced", that is, as open and inclusive as possible. The committee membership is expected to include ethnic, gender, and geographic diversity, as well as people with recognized expertise and judgment in a specific field, such as clinicians and researchers. Most members of the FDA's drug advisory committees are physician-scientists whose specialties and research involve the kinds of products being reviewed. Other members might include statisticians, epidemiologists, nutritionists, and toxicologists, experts in pre-clinical (animal) studies. The FDA also insists on getting industry and public perspectives, and nearly all committees include industry and consumer representation.

"Placing people on committees that have different perspectives and expertise gives balance to the discussions and final recommendations," says Linda Ann Sherman, M.D., M.P.A., former director of the FDA's Advisory Committee Oversight and Management Staff. "The agency aims for a lively discussion."

The industry representatives address global concerns for the industry. They do not represent their employers, rather, they bring their opinion of an issue like whether an additional preclinical study is necessary for a new class of drugs. The industry representative may express the opinion that the cost of such a study would be prohibitive and might not offer enough additional information to be cost-effective and could potentially delay the marketing of a product.

Consumers are represented on the committees by technically qualified professionals who have specific links with consumer advocacy groups. In addition, some committees have patient representatives. These individuals present "real world" concerns of the patient who is to be the potential recipient of the new medical product.

For example, scientists and the FDA might be considering a pill form of a drug that's already approved as an injection, but there may be problems with a person's ability to absorb the drug in pill form. The patient representative's role might be to point out that the committee should weigh the seriousness of the absorption problem against the value of patients taking the drug more consistently when it's offered in a more convenient dosage form. In any case, patient representatives, who can either be voting or non-voting members offer their experiences in an effort to provide a realistic look at a new product. It's important for patient representatives to have a general knowledge of the disease and the ability to comprehend the scientific data that are presented.

Most committee members vote at the end of each meeting on questions that are posed to them while some do not vote at all. The main impact of the member is their contribution to the discussion and not the final vote.

The notices requesting nominations to advisory committees are published in the Federal Register. Typically, the potential members are referred by professional, scientific and medical societies, academic institutions, government agencies, consumer and patient groups, and former and current advisory committee members. Sometimes, self-nominations also are encouraged.

The committees are required to dedicate a minimum of 60 minutes of each meeting to "open public comment." The public is invited to appear before the committee. Interested people may present information, orally or in writing, relevant to the meeting topic. Those who want to speak are encouraged to register.

Most meetings are supplemented by temporary voting members or consultants, who are the world's experts on the topic being discussed. These consultants are also special government employees but are present only for the specific meeting.

Committee Meetings

Committees, which range in size from 10 to 15 members (and may be supplemented by additional FDA consultants), typically meet twice a year in the Washington, D.C., area. The meetings generally last two days. An FDA official serves as the administrative executive secretary of each committee. Before an advisory committee meets, members would have already received and reviewed specific questions from the FDA along with other materials such as summaries of information on the safety and effectiveness of a new product. Prior to every meeting, each member is evaluated for any potential conflicts of interest. For example, a member may not participate in a meeting if he or she holds a financial interest in the product under consideration since the action taken could potentially provide the member with a personal financial gain or loss.

So, how does the agency determine which products will undergo an advisory committee review in the first place?

"Surprisingly," Sherman says, "many products do not make it to advisory committees." Those that do usually represent a new technology or some element of controversy.

For example, a meeting to discuss the latest data regarding silicone breast implant safety highlighted the mixed opinions about the risks and benefits of the implants. "The meeting provided a valuable forum for discussing the issue from many diverse perspectives and for raising important additional questions," Linda Kahan, deputy director of the FDA's Center for Devices and Radiological Health, said. "That is the point of the FDA's advisory committee process," she says, "to air issues that are controversial, complex, and do not have simple answers."

The decision to involve an advisory committee is usually at the discretion of the division director in one of the FDA's five product centers.

Sherman says, no count can be given to the number of products approved as a result of advisory committee recommendations. "Much of the advice accepted is not whether or not a product should be approved, but about some unique aspect of safety, effectiveness, or clinical development of that product."

In addition to serving as an important mechanism for outside input for the FDA, advisory committees are a vital public resource for information about new medical products. These meetings often represent the FDA's first public discussion of a new medical product and can be an invaluable source of information for patients, health care providers, and others who are interested in the product. Transcripts of FDA advisory committee discussions are posted at www.fda.gov/ohrms/dockets/ac/acmenu.htm

Each FDA committee must be renewed by the agency every two years, or its charter automatically expires. Renewals must be approved by the FDA commissioner or a designated appointing official. An assessment to renew is made based on the activity of the committee and the agency's continuing need for expertise in a particular scientific specialty.

"The FDA values the service its advisory committee members provide and the process itself," adds Sherman. "The system allows for the full participation of all of FDA's stakeholders to assist in the agency's regulatory decisions."

QUESTIONS

1. Write the principles involved in investigational use of drugs.

2. Classify investigational use of drugs.

3. Explain the role of a pharmacist in investigational use of drugs.

4. Explain the role of the Advisory Committee.

5. Describe the investigational use of drugs.

CHAPTER 21

INTERPRETATION OF CLINICAL LABORATORY TESTS

LEARNING OBJECTIVE

This chapter enlightens an important aspect of clinical practice - the diagnostic and monitoring tests conducted on a patient. How to interpret the complex results obtained by such tests are enumerated here hence the students will find it useful, during his carrier. That is the learning objective of the chapter.

PATIENT DATA

This is the data collected from the clinical laboratory tests carried out on a patient. It is very useful in the diagnosis, prevention, and treatment of diseases. However, in order to arrive at a decision, a reference standard is essential. This reference is usually available in the form of the quantitative range which is obtained by testing normal, disease-free individuals. While interpreting this data, one has to be careful as they do not always reflect the true condition of the patient. If the data indicates an excess of the range, it does not mean the person has got a disease. Similarly, if it is lower than the range, it is also not an indication of any serious problem with the patient. All this data has to be reviewed along with other signs and symptoms. There are many individual variables like age, sex, weight, body mass, disease, etc., that affect the results of these laboratory tests. Hence, a series of tests are to be carried out before arriving at a conclusion and to eliminate errors.

Need for Interpretation of Data

The main duty of a clinical pharmacist is to individualize the dose and drug regimen of the patient for which they have to rely upon the pharmacokinetic data as well as routine hematological data. Hence, they should at least possess a working knowledge of the significance of lab tests. Using that knowledge, they have to evaluate the outcome of the treatment given so far and recommend the changes to be made in the drugs, doses or treatment itself.

Additionally, depending on these results, they have to determine the appropriateness of the treatment, the efficacy of the treatment and also the drug's toxic effect, if any. Thus, the interpretation of clinical laboratory tests plays a major role in safe and effective therapy.

Fluid and Electrolytes Balance

Fluid and electrolytes are the important components of any living organism and they have to be in constant concentration and in balance for the body to function properly. The self-regulatory, feedback-controlled stabilization of the body as a whole or any subsystem like fluid and electrolytes balance is known as Homeostasis. [Homeo – of similarity, Stasis – stopping the flow]. Water or fluid, electrolytes, and acid-base balance are interrelated and the kidney plays an important role in their balance.

We will discuss a few important questions in this chapter like what disturbs their balance, what happens when they are in excess or lack and the steps to be taken to restore their balance, etc.

Water: The human body has a lot of water, that is, up to 50 to 60% of total body weight is water. It is required to maintain body temperature and in metabolic reactions. It is important to carry solutes from one part of our body to another part of our body. It is distributed as intercellular fluid [ICF] and extracellular fluid [ECF] at the ratio of 2:1. That is, about 28 liter of water is present in ICF and 14 liters in ECF. The ECF is further classified into interstitial fluids [10.5 lit] and intravascular fluid or plasma [3.5 lit]. The body regulates this balance by controlling water input and output.

Regulation of water intake: Depending on the climate and habit, we drink 0.5 to 5 lit of water per day. This apart, our solid food also contains some water. Together, they are called exogenous water and are mainly controlled by the thirst center present in the hypothalamus. It is stimulated whenever the water level in our body goes below the optimum level. Some amount of water is produced in our body itself by metabolic reactions, which is known as endogenous water and about 100 ml is produced in this manner.

Regulation of water output: Water is excreted by kidney via urine, skin via sweat, lungs via exhaled air, and G.I tract through feces. Out of these four, urine is the major source of elimination of water. About 1 to 2 liter of urine is excreted every day and it is controlled by vasopressin or antidiuretic hormone [ADH] secreted by the pituitary gland. The secretion of this hormone, in turn, is regulated by the osmotic pressure of plasma. The skin excretes about 400 ml to 450 ml of water through sweating which depends on the climate [Temperature and Humidity]. The Lungs excrete water through exhaled air, almost the same amount as skin, i.e., 400 ml per day. The loss of water through the GI tract via feces is estimated to be around 150 ml per day and needless to mention, it becomes multiple folds in diarrhea. Excess or less water intake or output leads to over hydration or dehydration respectively.

Over hydration: It is the retention of water in the body due to excessive intake of water, kidney failure or abnormal production of antidiuretic hormone [ADH]. This may lead to headaches and even convulsions. It is treated with a hypertonic saline solution and a complete stoppage of water intake until the patient recovers.

Dehydration: It is common in excess of loss of fluid during diarrhea, dysentery, and Cholera. There is loss of water from the body after fire accident [burns] and in excess vomiting or sweating. Usually, in these conditions, not only the body water is lost but also the electrolytes Na+, K+, etc. Dehydration is characterized by less urine output, shrunken cells of body due to excretion of water even from intercellular space and increased protein destruction. The protein and urea concentrations are thus increased in the blood. The clinical symptoms of dehydration are low B.P, increased pulse, sunken eye balls, etc. Usually, dehydration is treated with oral rehydration salt [ORS] where plenty of water is given orally. If it is not possible for any reason, 5% glucose or Normal Saline or Glucose Saline injections are given intravenously.

ELECTROLYTES

Electrolytes are inorganic salts which undergo dissolution and exist as positively and negatively charged ions in the animal body. For example, Sodium Chloride dissociate in to Na+ [cation] and Cl- [anion]. They are measured in milliequivalents [mEq/l]. The number of grams of a substance required to combine or displace one gram of hydrogen is known as milliequivalents weight and it's the one-thousandth part is also known as milliequivalents. It is calculated by the following formula:

$$mEq_1 = \frac{\text{mg per liter} \times \text{valency}}{\text{Atomic weight}}$$

To maintain osmotic and water balance, electrolytes are well-distributed in body fluids. As the electrolytes are in the form anion and cation, they have to be in equilibrium to maintain electrical neutrality.

To describe the electrolyte balance, we need to understand terms like osmolarity and osmolality which are used to explain the concentration of these molecules. Osmolarity is about moles or millimoles of electrolytes per liter of solution. On the other hand, osmolality measure the solute present in a fluid. It is defined as moles or millimoles per kg of solvent. If the solvent is pure water, there is no difference between osmolarity and osmolality. However, body fluids are not pure water and have a lot of constituents like proteins. Hence, osmolality is invariably used to describe the concentration of molecules.

The electrolytes are important for the proper functioning of the cells. They have to be balanced in both ECF and ICF because the ratio between them is important. Though this ratio is critical, its mechanism is very complex. We mainly study the concentration of electrolyte in plasma but to get a true picture, we need to dive deep in ancillary studies as well. For example, certain electrolytes like calcium and phosphate are present in hard tissues like bone and teeth.

The Osmolality of Plasma, ECF and ICF

Electrolytes are not equally distributed between ECF and ICF. For instance, Sodium is the major cation of ECF and chlorides and bicarbonates are its anion. On the other hand, Potassium is the predominant cation of ICF, phosphates, and sulphates are its anions. Only water moves freely between cells but for the electrolytes, an active transport mechanism is required for the movement between cells. Though electrolyte concentration differs between ECF and ICF, their osmolarity is equal.

The osmolality of plasma is measured by osmometer and it ranges from 285 to 295 milliosmoles per kg. Sodium and its anions are the major contributors [up to 90%] for this osmolality of plasma.

Balancing Electrolytes

Electrolytes are mainly balanced by three hormones, Aldosterone, Antidiuretic hormone, and Renin-angiotensin, and also by food intake. Aldosterone increases sodium reabsorption which increases the osmolality of plasma. This, in turn, stimulates the hypothalamus to release ADH which increases water reabsorption. Thus, all these hormones are interrelated and function in coordination to maintain normal fluid and electrolyte balance. Rennin angiotensin regulates the flow of aldosterone in this complex process.

Our body requirement of electrolytes is usually met by a balanced diet. During summer, we may need to support our bodies with extra electrolytes. The normal range of these electrolytes and water are given in the following Table

Table 21.1 Normal Values of Electrolytes

Electrolytes	In serum	In urine
Sodium	135 -155 mEq/L	150 – 197 mEq/ day
Potassium	3.9 -5.6 mEq/L	20 -64 mEq/ day
Calcium	8.8 -10.2 mEq/L	--
Chloride	95 – 106 mEq/L	180 – 270 mEq/day
Total anions	154 mEq/L	--
Total cations	154 mEq/L	--

Estimation of Electrolytes

Body fluids are analyzed for the estimation of electrolytes using various instrumental methods. The flame photometry, x-ray fluorescence, Atomic absorption spectrometry, and colorimetric techniques are used in the identification and estimation of anions and cations in the body fluids. The recent advanced methods determine both anions and cations simultaneously. Normally, sodium and potassium in serum are estimated either by Flame photometry or specific Atomic absorption spectrometry. Chloride is determined potentiometrically using silver-silver chloride pH electrodes. Calcium in urine or serum is estimated by EDTA method of analysis, Atomic absorption spectroscopy, or Flame photometry. Magnesium is measured by ion-specific electrode and trace elements like copper, zinc, and iron are determined by flame photometric or colorimetric methods.

Uses of Study of Electrolyte Balance

The study of electrolyte balances is a useful indicator of renal and cardiac failure, anuria, adrenal cortical insufficiency and excess of electrolyte excretion. The pancreatic cystic fibrosis is detected by an excess of chloride ions in the perspiration of patients. Thus, the study of electrolyte and water balance is useful as a valuable diagnostic tool. As the analysis of metabolic excretion rates is carried out in these studies, it is useful to evaluate the functions of various organs like liver, kidney, thyroid and other glands.

Disturbance of Electrolyte Balance

Severe excess or lack of electrolytes in the body leads to various disorders and diseases. They are indicated by many clinical symptoms and are often treatable. The causes of the disturbed balance of electrolytes are many and outside the preview of this chapter. However, a clinical pharmacist is concerned with the effect of drugs which may be the reason for such conditions.

Let us take a look at the table below to understand that.

Table 21.2 Effect of Drugs on Electrolytes Balance

Condition	Sodium	Potassium	Calcium	Phosphates
Excess	Hypernatraemia	Hyperkalaemia	Hypercalcaemia	Hyperphosphataemia
Symptoms	Muscle weakness, confusion, etc	Asymptomatic but fatal	Seen in Malignancy and Renal transplantation	Seen in renal failure, Hypo para thyroidis
Possible causative drugs for excess	Phenytoin, Methyl Dopa, oral Contraceptives, Clonidine, Corticosteroid, etc	Digoxin, Isoniazid, Tetracycline, NSAID, Cyclosporine, Penicillin, etc	Lithium, Tamoxifen, Diuretics, etc	All drugs causing kidney damage
Less [Deficient]	Hyponatraemia	Hypokalaemia	Hypocalcaemia	Hypophosphataemia
Symptoms	Nausia, Confusion, Drowsiness, etc	Muscle weakness, Hypotonia, Depression, Confusion, etc	Seen in Pancreatitis, Liver disease, Kidney disease, Vitamin D deficiency, etc	Muscle weakness
Possible drugs responsible for deficiency	Diuretics, Heparin, NSAID, Tolbutamide, Amphotericin, Miconazole, etc	Aspirin, Corticosteroids, Gentamicin, Insulin, Laxatives, Salicylates, etc	Phenytoin, Phenobarbitone, Aminoglycosides, Furasimide, etc	All drugs causing kidney damage

Haematology Data

Among the tests performed on a patient, the blood test is the one that helps the physician more than any other test. The characters of blood cells and other components give the first line of diagnostic features about the diseases, deficiencies or defects that affect the human body. Hence, a clinical pharmacist must be thorough with these tests.

1. **RBC count:** The normal range of Red Blood Cells in males is 4.4 to 6.1 × 1012/L and 4.0 to 5.5 × 1012/L in females. If it is less, the condition is called anemia and the excess of it is known as hypoxia. Anemia may be microcytic due to iron deficiency or macrocytic due to folic acid and vitamin B12 deficiency.

2. **Reticulocyte count:** It should be 0.5% to 1% of RBC. In hemorrhage and hemolysis, it goes up to 40% of RBC. The reticulocyte count is useful to evaluate the response of bone marrow to iron, foliate, vitamin B12 therapy.

3. **Mean Cell Volume (MCV):** It is an average volume of a single red cell. It is measured in Femtolitres (10–15 L). If the MCV is low, it is known as microcytic MCV and if it is high, we call it macrocytic MCV. The former MCV is due to deficiency of iron and the latter is due to folic acid deficiency.

4. **Packed Cell Volume (PCV):** It is the ratio of the volume occupied by red cells to the total volume of blood. The normal value is 45%. Nowadays, it is calculated by multiplying MCV and RBC. PCV is decreased in anemia, and hemorrhage, whereas it is increased in polycythemia. Furthermore, it is altered in macrocytosis and microcytosis.

5. **Mean Cell Haemoglobin Concentration (MCHC):** It is a measure of the average concentration of Haemoglobin in 100 ml of red cells. It is measured in grams/lit or as a percentage. The normal value is 315 to 345 g/L. If it is low, iron deficiency anemia is the reason and if it is on a higher side, severe, prolonged dehydration is indicated.

6. **Hemoglobin:** It is one of the important measurements in blood tests. It differs, depending on sex. The men have more Haemoglobin than women due to the presence of more RBC and menstrual loss, respectively. The normal value of men is 13.5 to 17 g/dl and a woman is 11.5 to 16.5 g/dl. Values less than these indicate anemia.

7. **Platelets (Thrombocytes):** It is formed in the bone marrow. If it is synthesized less in the bone marrow or destructed after formation, a lesser number is seen in the blood analysis. As it has a short life of only 8 to 12 days, it is easy to evaluate drug-induced thrombocytopenia (less number). It comes back to the normal level once the drug is stopped. The lesser number of platelet may also be due to pregnancy, viral infection or bleeding. An increased number is seen in Malignancy and inflammatory diseases. The normal value of the platelet is 150 to 450 ×109/l.

8. **White Blood Cells (Leucocytes):** This is one of the very important blood components and its character and count in blood tests reveal a lot of information about the condition of the patient. There are two types of WBC, namely Granulocytes and Agranulocytes (Lymphocytes). Granulocytes are further sub-divided into monocytes and polymorphonuclear granulocytes which consist of Neutrophil, Basophil, and Eosinophil. Usually, WBC is measured and reported as Total Count (TC) and as differential Count (DC) which lists various types of polymorphonuclear granulocytes.

   (a) **Neutrophils:** They form the majority of white cells. The normal range is from 50% to 70% of total white blood cells. If it is more, there may be inflammation or tissue damage in patients. On the other hand, if it is less, it indicates malignancy or hepatitis.

(b) Basophils: They are less than 1% of white cells. Their function is not clear. However, they are found less in malignancy conditions.

(c) Eosinophils: The normal value of Eosinophil is less than 6% of TC. It is increased in allergic conditions like asthma, hay fever, drug sensitivity, and malignant diseases.

(d) Monocytes: They form 0% to 7% of total white cells. They are increased in infections like TB, typhoid, etc.

(e) Lymphocytes: They are mainly found in spleen and other lymphatic tissue. However, they are present in large numbers next to neutrophils in the blood. The normal value is 20% to 40%, but they increase in viral infections like infectious hepatitis, decreased in AIDS, renal failure, and cardiac failure.

9. **Erythrocyte Sedimentation Rate (ESR):** ESR is a measure of sedimentation rate of red cells in a sample of blood containing an anticoagulant over a period of one hour in a cylindrical tube. Its normal value is less than 10 mm/hr. It is increased in rheumatoid arthritis, inflammatory bowel diseases, malignancies, and infections.

10. **Bleeding time:** It is the time taken by the blood to stop bleeding from the wound. It shows the hemostatic efficiency of the blood. Normally, the blood should stop within 2 to 5 minutes. It is increased in thrombocytopenia, platelet disorders and prolonged use of aspirin and anticoagulants. Hence, the clinical pharmacists should take care of these conditions in the patient.

11. **Whole blood clotting time:** It is the time taken by the blood to clot when tested outside the body (in vitro). The normal range is 4 to 9 minutes at 37°C. A prolonged time indicates hemophilia, factor 8 deficiencies or presence of anticoagulants.

12. **Prothrombin Time (PT):** It is the time required to clot citrated plasma to which an optimum amount of thromboplastin and calcium has been added. The usual prothrombin time is 12 to 15 seconds. The PT is usually indicated in the form of a ratio known as International Normalized Ratio (INR) which is the ratio of PT of the patient and the normal (disease-free) man. The result of oral anticoagulant therapy can be monitored using the PT. Also, it is useful to evaluate liver function.

13. **Blood sugar:** The blood sugar level is an important parameter that is usually checked for patients. A fasting blood glucose level of 70 to 110 mg/dl is considered normal. It is usually increased in diabetes. However, it cannot be confirmed by this elevation alone as other conditions like severe nephritis, pancreatic disease, hyperthyroidism, and certain liver diseases also increase blood sugar levels. Hence, the glucose tolerance test [GTT] should be done in suspected cases. Around 50 gm of glucose is given to the patient. The blood sugar level reaches the maximum within a short while and should return to normal within 1hour 30 minutes to 2 hours. If not, and more than 50% in excess of the fasting sugar level is there diabetes is confirmed. Similarly, low sugar levels indicate hypopituitarism, cretinism or hypothyroidism.

14. **Serum enzymes:** Alkaline Phosphate ALP (or) AP: It is present in liver, bone, intestinal wall and placenta. Each of the above sites produces a specific isoenzyme of AP. The

normal range of AP is 30 to 90 IU/L. It is increased in jaundice, osteomalacia, rickets, and in low absorption of vitamin D and calcium. It is decreased in the low phosphate conditions of the body.

15. **Creatine Phosphokinase: (CPK) or Creatin Kinase (CK):** This enzyme is found in heart muscle, skeletal muscle, and brain tissue. There are three isoenzymes of CPK known as CPK-MM found in the skeletal muscle, CPK-BB in the brain tissue and CPK-MB in the heart muscle. The measurement of these enzymes indicates the source of damage. Usually, CPK-MM isozyme is present in serum. The CPK levels are increased in tissue damage conditions like falling, vigorous exercise, deep IM injection, etc. The diagnosis of acute myocardial infarction is possible by measurement of the CPK level.

16. **Lactic acid Dehydrogenase: (LDH or LD):** This enzyme interconvert lactate and pyruvate in the body and present in all the metabolizing cells. There are five isoenzymes of LDH, namely LDH 1 to LDH 5. Out of these, the first two are present in the heart, third in the lungs, fourth and fifth in the liver and skeletal muscles respectively. The measurement of these enzymes point out where the damage is and this helps in the diagnosis of myocardial infarction, liver, and lung diseases.

URINALYSIS

Urine analysis is one of the major routine analyses done in any clinical laboratory. It gives valuable data to treating physicians for diagnosing and determining the line of treatment and to modify the existing treatment. Other advantages include the easy collection of the sample of the urine from the patients with no instrument requirement, as seen for other samples.

The following are some important tests done on the urine:

1. Physical properties of urine

2. Identification of normal inorganic constituents

3. Identification of normal organic constituents

4. Estimation of glucose

5. Estimation of calcium

6. Estimation of Diastase and

7. Estimation of creatinine

All of the above tests give useful data to determine the disorder or disease of the patient.

1. **Physical properties:** In this test, the volume, color, turbidity, specific gravity, odor, and pH are verified. The volume of more than 1500 ml per day indicates polyurea and less than 1000 ml indicates dehydration, fever, diarrhea or vomiting. Similarly, yellowish-green to brown color of urine may be due to jaundice and dirty blue indicates cholera or typhus. When the odor of urine is unpleasant and aromatic, it denotes microbial decomposition and if it is a sweet odor, ketosis is suspected. The acidic or alkaline pH of urine may be due to acidosis or alkalosis.

2. **Inorganic constituents:** If the decreased amount of chlorides are found in urine, fever, nephritis, and diarrhea are indicated. The excess of phosphates is seen in certain bone diseases and the decreased amount is seen in hypoparathyroidism. Similarly, the excess of sulphate in urine denotes the breakdown of tissue protein.

3. **Organic constituents:** Urea, uric acid, and creatinine are the normal organic constituents of urine. They are tested by simple chemical tests for their presence. But a quantitative analysis is carried out using calorimeter and other instruments. The excess or lack of these organic constituents point out to some underlying problems.

The other organic constituents of the urine are protein, glucose, ketone, pigments, and blood. Each one of it, if found or exceed the normal value denotes some disease. For example, the excess of glucose indicates diabetes mellitus and ketone indicates excessive oxidation of fatty acids, starvation, or fasting. If Bilrubine appears in the urine, obstructive jaundice is suspected and urochromogen is due to tuberculosis. The appearance of blood in urine is known as Haematuria. It could be indicating towards lesions in kidney, tuberculosis, cancer or renal stone.

4. **Estimation of calcium:** It is estimated to study diseases of parathyroid and kidney. Urine calcium is in excess in hypoparathyroidism and stone formation. It is decreased in many cases of nephrosis and acute nephritis.

5. **Estimation of Diastase:** The enzyme diastase converts starch into maltose. The excess or lack of diastase in urine points to the disorders like duodenal ulcer, pancreatitis, and intestinal obstructions.

6. **Estimation of Creatinine:** Creatinine is the waste product of creatine metabolism. If it appears in the urine, it is known as creatinuria. Its value exceeds in fever, starvation, and in diabetes. It is estimated using photoelectric calorimeter by measuring the optical density.

It is clear from the above tests that simple urinalysis helps the physician in a significant way in the clinical practice.

Students are advised to refer to standard books on Biochemistry and clinical pathology for normal values of urine constituents and also for the test procedure.

QUESTIONS

1. Write a note on disturbance of electrolyte balance.

2. List the methods of estimation of electrolytes.

3. What are the tests done on Urine?

4. Explain the significance of estimating WBC and its types.

5. Describe the tests and interpret the results of Urinalysis.

REFERENCE BOOKS

1. Remington's 'Pharmaceutical Sciences'. 18th edition.

2. 'Hospital Pharmacy' by Willian E. Hassan. 4th edition.

3. 'Clinical Pharmacy and Hospital Drug Management' by David H. Lawson and Michael E. Richard.

4. Oxford's 'Textbook of Clinical Pharmacology and Drug Therapy, by D. S. Graham Smith and J. K. Armson.

5. 'Clinical Pharmacokinetics Concepts and Applications' by Malcolm Rowland and Thomas N. Tozer.

6. British National Formulary.

7. 'Textbook of Biopharmaceutics and Clinical Pharmacokinetics' by Sartaray Hiage.

8. 'The Pharmacological Basis of Therapeutics' edited by Louis S. Goodmann and Alfred Gilmann.

9. 'Clinical Pharmacokinetics and TDM' Article by S.B. Bhise, et al., IJPE, Sept, 1998.

10. 'A Textbook of Hospital Pharmacy' by S.H. Merchant and J.S. Qadry.

11. 'Biopharmaceutics and Clinical Pharmacokinetics' by Gibaldi M. 4th edition.

12. 'Basic Clinical Pharmacokinetics' by Winter M.E.

13. 'Avery's Drug Treatment' 3rd Edition – edited by Trevor M. Speight.

14. 'Textbook of Therapeutics' by Herfindal and Gourley – 6th edition.

15. 'Materials Management' by C.B. Agarwal.

16. 'Pharmaceutical Practice' by Richard and Winfeild.

17. 'Medical Pharmacology' by K.D. Thirupathi.

18. 'A Textbook of Clinical Pharmacy Practice' edited by G. Parthasarathi, et al.

19. 'Clinical Pharmacy and Therapeutics' by Roger Walker et al., 4th edition.

20. 'Remington: The Science and Practice of Pharmacy' 19th Edition & 22nd Edition.

21. 'The Merck Manual'– 15th edition. MSD Research Lab, N.J.

22. 'Pharmacist's Drug Hand Book' –American Society of Health System Pharmacists.

23. 'Clinical Pharmacy and Therapeutics' 4th Edition – Eric T. Herfindal, et al, Wolters Kluwer, NY.

24. 'Biochemistry' 4th Edition – U. Satyanarayana, et al, Elsevier.

25. 'Practical Manual of Biochemistry and Clinical Pathology' – G. D. Gupta, et al 4th Edition, Nirali Prakashan.

26. 'Principles of Pharmacology', 4th Edition,-- David. E. Golan , et al, Wolters Kluwer, USA

27. 'A Guide to G.D practitioners'- WHO.

REFERENCE WEBSITES

1. www.who.int

2. www.ncbi.nlm.nih.gov

3. www.mun.ca

4. www.fda.gov

5. www.ajhp.org

6. www.en.wikipedia.org

7. www.student.bmj.com

8. www.lifetechnologies.com

9. www.medilexicon.com

10. http://quizlet.com

11. http://.nih.gov